THE NEUROHYPOPHYSIS

Physiological and Clinical Aspects

THE NEUROHYPOPHYSIS

Physiological and Clinical Aspects

Edited by
Seymour Reichlin, M.D., Ph.D.

Tufts-New England Medical Center
Boston, Massachusetts

PLENUM MEDICAL BOOK COMPANY
NEW YORK AND LONDON

Library of Congress Cataloging in Publication Data

Main entry under title:

The Neurohypophysis, physiological and clinical aspects.

Includes bibliographical references and index.
1. Neurohypophysis — Diseases. 2. Neurohypophysis. I. Reichlin, Seymour. [DNLM:
1. Pituitary gland, Posterior — Congresses. 2. Neurophysins — Congresses. 3. Pituitary
diseases — Congresses. WK 520 N4946]
RC658.N48   1984   616.4'7   84-4861
ISBN-13: 978-1-4684-4738-5   e-ISBN-13: 978-1-4684-4736-1
DOI: 10.1007/978-1-4684-4736-1

© 1984 Plenum Publishing Corporation
Softcover reprint of the hardcover 1st edition 1984
233 Spring Street, New York, N.Y. 10013

Plenum Medical Book Company is an imprint of Plenum Publishing Corporation

CONTRIBUTORS

H. Franklin Bunn   Hematology Division, Department of Medicine, Brigham and Women's Hospital, Harvard Medical School, Boston, Massachusetts 02115

William E. Cobb   Division of Endocrinology and Metabolism, Department of Medicine, Tufts–New England Medical Center Hospital, Boston, Massachusetts 02111

Walter Davis   Department of Microscopic Anatomy, Baylor College of Dentistry, Dallas, Texas 75246

Franklin H. Epstein   Charles A. Dana Research Institute, Harvard–Thorndike Laboratory, and Department of Medicine, Beth Israel Hospital, Harvard Medical School, Boston, Massachusetts 02115

Harold Gainer   Section on Functional Neurochemistry, Laboratory of Neurochemistry and Neuroimmunology, National Institute of Child Health and Human Development, National Institutes of Health, Bethesda, Maryland 20205

David B. P. Goodman   Department of Pathology and Laboratory Medicine, University of Pennsylvania Medical School, Philadelphia, Pennsylvania 19104

Susan Hou   Department of Internal Medicine, St. Margaret's Hospital for Women, Boston, Massachusetts 02125; and Department of Medicine, Tufts University School of Medicine, Boston, Massachusetts 02111

Anna Hou-Yu   Department of Neurology, College of Physicians and Surgeons, Columbia University, New York, New York 10032

Kalman Kovacs   Department of Pathology, St. Michael's Hospital, and University of Toronto, Toronto, Ontario M5B 1W8, Canada

Jeanne M. Lusher   Children's Hospital of Michigan, Detroit, Michigan 48201

Arnold M. Moses   Veterans Administration Medical Center and Department of Medicine, State University of New York, Upstate Medical Center, Syracuse, New York 13210

Gajanan Nilaver   Department of Neurology, College of Physicians and Surgeons, Columbia University, New York, New York 10032

Seymour Reichlin   Division of Endocrinology, Department of Medicine, Tufts–New England Medical Center, Boston, Massachusetts 02111

Alan G. Robinson   University of Pittsburgh School of Medicine, Pittsburgh, Pennsylvania 15261

Robert M. Rosa   Charles A. Dana Research Institute, Harvard–Thorndike Laboratory, and Department of Medicine, Beth Israel Hospital, Harvard Medical School, Boston, Massachusetts 02115

Ann-Judith Silverman   Department of Anatomy and Cell Biology, College of Physicians and Surgeons, Columbia University, New York, New York 10032

A. Indira Warrier   Children's Hospital of Michigan, Detroit, Michigan 48201

Earl A. Zimmerman   Department of Neurology, College of Physicians and Surgeons, Columbia University, New York, New York 10032

PREFACE

The elucidation of the structure, function, and clinical significance of the neurohypophysis has been one of the most rewarding chapters in the history of endocrinology. Diabetes insipidus, which can be manifested by passage of 15 liters of urine a day, is one of the most dramatic disorders of the endocrine system, and can readily be managed by replacement therapy with the natural secretions of this gland, or with synthetic analogues that provide a more favorable therapeutic ratio. The neurohypophysis is the archetypical neurosecretory gland. Its secretions arise within well defined nerve cells in the hypothalamus, are transported by axoplasmic flow to nerve endings in the neural lobe, are released in response to propagated action potentials, and are regulated by neurotransmitters and osmotic signals. This gland is a model for homeostatic regulation; functional disorders of this regulation lead to well defined disorders such as the syndrome of inappropriate secretion of antidiuretic hormone (SIADH), which can be mimicked by the ectopic secretion of its hormones by tumor cells. These hormones were the first peptides to be sequenced and synthesized chemically and their structure–function relations have been characterized as well as those of any of the peptide hormones. The concept that peptide hormones generally arise as products of the processing of a larger prohormone precursor was first developed from studies of the neurohypophysis. The concept of stimulus–secretion coupling was first applied in neuronal tissue to the neurohypophysis.

For these and many other reasons, the neurohypophysis has received an enormous amount of attention from neural scientists, clinicians, and endocrinologists. It is surprising therefore that a comprehensive summary of the current status of knowledge of the neurohypophysis in a form that would be useful to investigators and clinicians has not been published.

This monograph seeks to fill that need. It is based on a conference on the neurohypophysis that was held in Boston in 1982 under the sponsorship of the Tufts University School of Medicine, but the individual chapters have, for the most part, been expanded by their contributors in order to broaden the coverage of their areas. Two of the participants in this conference discussed the use of vasopressin and its long-acting analogue 1-desamino-8-D-arginine vasopressin (dDAVP) in the novel treatment of sickle cell anemia and von Willebrand's disease—two nonendocrine disorders depending upon the action of antidiuretic hormone to reduce serum osmolarity and to mobilize the release of Factor VIII, respectively. In addition, a chapter on SIADH has been added.

We have sought in this volume to provide both a comprehensive monograph, useful as a reference volume to investigators, and a textbook for students and clinicians.

Seymour Reichlin

Boston

CONTENTS

Chapter 6

Pathology of the Neurohypophysis 95

Kalman Kovacs

Chapter 7

Clinical and Laboratory Features of Central and Nephrogenic
Diabetes Insipidus and Primary Polydipsia 115

Arnold M. Moses

Chapter 8

Management of Neurogenic Diabetes Insipidus with dDAVP and
Other Agents 139

William E. Cobb

Chapter 9

Syndrome of Inappropriate Antidiuretic Hormone Secretion   165

Susan Hou

Chapter 10

Treatment of Sickle Cell Anemia with dDAVP   191

Franklin H. Epstein, Robert M. Rosa, and H. Franklin Bunn

Chapter 11

dDAVP in von Willebrand's Disease and in Moderately Severe

Jeanne M. Lusher and A. Indira Warrier

THE
NEUROHYPOPHYSIS

THE NEUROHYPOPHYSIS
Historical Overview

Seymour Reichlin

We owe the beginning of our understanding of the function of the neurohypophysis to the pioneering work of two clinicians, Farini and von den Velden, and to the concept of neurosecretion pioneered by an anatomist, Ernst Scharrer. As detailed by Heller,[1] the antidiuretic effects of extracts of the neurohypophysis were first demonstrated by Farini, assistant physician in the medical division of the Ospedale Civile in Venice (reported in 1913) and von den Velden, *Oberarzt* in the medical clinic of Düsseldorf (also reported in 1913). The "establishment" view of the neurohypophysis at the turn of the century was that it functioned to regulate blood pressure, because both increased and decreased blood pressure had been recorded following injections of neural lobe extracts. It was also believed to be a gland that promoted diuresis, because injection of neural lobe extracts stimulated urine flow in anesthetized dogs. Independently of one another, the two clinicians had come to the conclusion on the basis of autopsy findings in patients dying with diabetes insipidus that this disease was a deficiency disorder caused by lack of function of the neural lobe. Farini reported on two cases "whose daily urine volume of 5–6 and 7.5–8 liters respectively" was decreased by injection of posterior pituitary extract. Von den Velden reported one patient whose urinary specific gravity rose from 1005 to 1010 and whose urine volume fell from 6 liters/24 hr to less than 3 liters/24 hr. He also showed an antidiuretic effect in two hydrated normal volunteers. Subsequently Starling and Verney reported in 1924 that the extract acted directly on the kidney to produce these

Seymour Reichlin • Division of Endocrinology, Department of Medicine, Tufts–New England Medical Center, Boston, Massachusetts 02111.

effects, and Verney later demonstrated the antidiuretic effect of saline perfusion of the carotid artery of the dog. From this finding he postulated the
existence of central nervous system osmoreceptors and showed the effect of
conditioning and emotional stress on antidiuretic hormone (ADH) secretion.
Verney's accomplishments in demonstrating neural control of the neurohypophysis were an important factor in arousing Geoffry Harris's interest in and
committment to the study of neural control of the anterior lobe of the pituitary.

   By the late 1930s the physiological basis of homeostatic control of water
balance by neurogenically mediated ADH release was well understood. In
the intervening years, the specific secretions of the neurohypophysis have
been isolated, chemically identified, synthesized chemically, and applied to
therapy. Assays for the hormones of the neural lobe have made it possible
to define in precise terms the nature of the control mechanism and its operation
in health and disease, and have led to the demonstration of many other
biologically active substances in the neurohypophysis. Most recently, the
mode of biosynthesis of the neurohypophysial hormones has been elucidated,
as have the structural relationships among vasopressin, oxytocin, their respective prohormones. The availability of antisera specific for the secretions
of the neurohypophysis have made possible the precise delineation of the
neural pathways that regulate ADH secretion and a physiological analysis of
the pathological lesions that affect this region.

   The other important factor that led to our understanding of neural lobe
function is the elucidation of the concept of neurosecretion. In this effort, the
neurohypophysis has served as the classical paradigm in the mammal. According to Bern and Knowles,[2] themselves pioneers in the field, the idea that
a nerve cell could also be a secretory cell was first put forth in 1919 by Carl
Speidel, who observed a population of giant neurons located in the posterior
spinal cord of elasmobranch fishes that "possessed all of the cytological
attributes associated with secretory activity." We now know that these cells
project to the urophysis, a neurohypophysislike structure in the tail region of
the fish, and that the secretion of this gland is urophysin, a linear peptide of
established structure. About a decade later, Ernst Scharrer made the observation that similar cells were present in the hypothalamus of fishes. In the
1930s, he and his wife Berta Scharrer and their co-worker Wolfgang Bargmann were to make the observations that have led to the now-general concept
of neurosecretion. The definition of *neurosecretion* has undergone many trans-
formations (see ref. 2 for discussion), but, in its most widely accepted form,
neurosecretion refers to the elaboration of secretory products by nerve cells

and their release as hormones into the bloodstream. Because an analogous process can occur with release of the secretory product as a neurotransmitter, i.e., in relation to a neuron or in relation to a glandular cell such as the salivary gland, a more general definition would regard neurosecretion as a property of virtually all neurons, namely the elaboration of specific secretory products that may act locally, or at a remote site.

In the case of the neurohypophysis, the neurosecretory basis of its function was recognized early by the Scharrers because the Gomori stain was very reactive with the cysteine-rich neurophysins. It was possible very early (because of the relatively easy access to this system) for Hild to show that a ligature on the neural stalk (or section of the stalk) led to proximal accumulation of secretory product, thus establishing the concept of axonal flow from cell body to axonal process. The relatively simple chemical structures of the secretions of the neurohypophysis, the nonapeptides vasopressin and oxytocin, made them accessible to the early technological methods of sequencing and chemical synthesis that were available to du Vigneaud and his colleagues in the 1950s and which won him a Nobel prize. Du Vigneaud's success in isolating and synthesizing biologically active peptides was a major spur to Guillemin and his school, and led to their remarkable success in structural identification of the hypophysiotropic peptides.

The power of the neurosecretory concept for modern neurobiology can hardly be exaggerated.[3-7] Neurosecretion has expanded the number of potential neurotransmitters and neuroregulators by more than an order of magnitude and has provided the essential link between the molecular biology of the endocrine system and that of the nervous system. An excellent example of these new insights is the finding (discussed in this volume by Zimmerman et al. in Chapter 2) that the paraventricular neurophysinergic and vasopressinergic neurons have an extensive distribution within the brain that is quite distinct from their neural lobe distribution. With few if any exceptions, all of the physiological and anatomical elements of neurosecretory systems within the brain are, as far as is known now, identical in basic plan with the neurons of the supraoptico- and paraventriculo-hypophysial systems.

Advances in understanding of the structure–function relationships of vasopressin have permitted the synthesis of high-potency analogues with minimal hypertensive action that are effective by intranasal insufflation. This agent has been used to induce a state of hemodilution, proven to be useful in the prophylaxis of recurrent attacks of sickle cell crises. An unexpected physiological action of vasopressin, its ability to mobilize the release of Factor

VIII, has led to its use in patients with several clotting disorders of the von Willebrand's type. For all these reasons and many others, the neurohypophysis has served biology superbly well as the classic model of neuroendocrine control of a homeostatic function. Diabetes insipidus has been a model example of a deficiency disease with an unambiguous pathophysiological basis and a rational basis for therapy.

REFERENCES

1. Heller H: History of neurohypophysial research, in Knobil E, Sawyer WH (eds): *Handbook of Physiology*, Section 7: *Endocrinology*. Washington, DC, American Physiological Society, 1974, pp 103–117.
2. Bern HA, Knowles FGW: Neurosecretion, in Martini L, Ganong WF (eds): *Neuroendocrinology*. New York, Academic Press, 1966, vol 1, pp 139–186.
3. Gainer H (ed): *Peptides in Neurobiology*. New York, Plenum Press, 1977.
4. Gotto AM Jr, Peck EJ Jr, Boyd AE III (eds): *Brain Peptides: A New Endocrinology*. Amsterdam, Elsevier/North Holland Biomedical Press, 1979.
5. Bloom F (ed): *Peptides: Integrators of Cell and Tissue Function*. New York, Raven Press, 1980.
6. Martin JB, Reichlin S, Bick KL (eds): *Neurosecretion and Brain Peptides*. New York, Raven Press, 1981.
7. Schmitt FO, Bird SJ, Bloom FE (eds): *Molecular Genetic Neuroscience*. New York, Raven Press, 1982.

2

ANATOMY OF PITUITARY AND EXTRAPITUITARY VASOPRESSIN SECRETORY SYSTEMS

Earl A. Zimmerman, Anna Hou-Yu, Gajanan Nilaver, and Ann-Judith Silverman

1. INTRODUCTION

1.1. Historical Overview

The well accepted concept of neurosecretion, namely that certain neurons produce biologically active peptides, was derived from pioneering studies of the hypothalamo-neurohypophysial system, which secretes vasopressin and oxytocin into the systemic circulation.[1,2] This neurosecretory system has been studied for nearly half a century.[3] Today it still is an important model for the understanding of other peptidergic neurons that are less accessible to study, including the smaller vasopressin and oxytocin neurons that project to regions outside the hypothalamus.[4] The organization of the system—with its large cell bodies located in the hypothalamus, projecting by a converging pathway in median eminence and pituitary stalk, and large stores of granules containing the hormones concentrated in posterior pituitary gland—has made the system

Earl A. Zimmerman, Anna Hou-Yu, and Gajanan Nilaver • Department of Neurology, College of Physicians and Surgeons, Columbia University, New York, New York 10032. Ann-Judith Silverman • Department of Anatomy and Cell Biology, College of Physicians and Surgeons, Columbia University, New York, New York 10032.

more accessible to anatomical,[2,4] biochemical,[5,6] and physiological[7,8] study than other neurosecretory systems, such as those producing releasing and inhibiting factors that regulate the anterior pituitary gland.

1.2. Studies with Gomori Stains

Although a neural connection between hypothalamus and posterior pituitary gland was suggested at the turn of the 20th century by classical anatomical techniques, this pathway was not fully established until midcentury, when Gomori stains were applied to the system.[1-3] The stains (aldehyde–fuchsin, chrome–alum–hematoxylin) were initially used to identify what turned out to be insulin-secreting B cells of the pancreas.[9] When applied to sections of the brain and pituitary, these stains reacted selectively with the large neuronal cell bodies (magnocellular) of the supraoptic and paraventricular nuclei of the hypothalamus.[1,3] Furthermore, beaded axonal pathways could be traced from these perikarya through the internal zone (zona interna) of the median eminence, down the pituitary stalk to end near blood vessels in the posterior pituitary gland. These studies not only defined the hypothalamo-neurohypophysial system anatomically, they also suggested that these neurons contained and presumably secreted a hormonal substance(s) at their terminals. Interruption of these fibers in the pituitary stalk caused a proximal buildup and distal loss of stainable neurosecretory material. This suggested that neurohypophysial principles, soon to be chemically identified as oxytocin and vasopressin by du Vigneaud and colleagues,[10] were produced in the cell bodies and transported to posterior pituitary by axonal flow. These findings dispelled the view that the pituicytes of the posterior pituitary gland, which are now known to be glial and lack neurosecretory granules, produced these hormones. The basis of the Gomori stain is primarily due to unusually high amounts of sulfhydryl groups in the neurophysin proteins associated with the hormones.[2] The Gomori stains can also react with disulfide groups in oxytocin and vasopressin, but they contribute far less than the neurophysins to staining.

In recent years, immunocytochemical studies using antisera to neurophysins have confirmed and extended the earlier results using Gomori stains, including the finding that some fibers projected to the portal capillary system of the median eminence[11] and even to extrahypothalamic sites.[12] The immunocytochemical methods[13,14] proved to be more sensitive as more cells were found, including some in the suprachiasmatic nucleus.[14] These had previously been missed totally, probably because of relatively low content of neurosecretory material. The newer methods were also more specific, particularly when antisera to the hormones and their related neurophysins were applied. Both oxytocin and vasopressin neurons were found in both the supraoptic and paraventricular nuclei,[14] contrary to earlier views based on bioassay and lesion studies,[15] which suggested that vasopressin was produced solely by the supraoptic nuclei and oxytocin exclusively by the paraventricular nuclei.

1.3. Biochemistry and Autoradiography

Studies of the hypothalamo-neurohypophysial system in the 1960s by autoradiographic and biochemical methods utilizing incorporation of [^{35}S]cystine[2,5] brought further confirmation and definition of the neurosecretory concept. It was shown that the hormones and associated neurophysins were synthesized by a ribosomal mechanism in the perikarya of the supraoptic and paraventricular nuclei, packaged into large granules in the Golgi apparatus, and transported by fast axonal transport to secretory terminals.[2,5,6] An exocytotic mechanism of secretion[16] was supported by evidence for cosecretion of neurophysin and vasopressin into the general circulation,[5] since both are highly concentrated in the posterior pituitary granules. Purification of the granules facilitated further biochemical characterization of the neurophysins, and it was eventually agreed that there were primarily two neurophysins, one associated with oxytocin and another with vasopressin, each weighing about 10,000 daltons.[6] Subsequent preparation of antisera to the neurophysins, as well as the hormones, not only permitted radioimmunoassay of these oligopeptides in blood, cerebrospinal fluid, and brain tissues (see Chapter 5), but also provided new anatomical probes for immunocytochemistry in the early 1970s.[14] These antisera also facilitated reinvestigation of the existence of a larger precursor molecule required for biosynthesis of vasopressin, for which initial evidence was provided by the pioneering work of Sachs et al.[5,17] Gainer and collaborators (see Chapter 3) have shown convincing evidence for two different precursors of approximately 20,000 daltons for oxytocin (pro-oxyphysin) and vasopressin (pro-pressophysin).[6] Homozygous Brattleboro rats manifesting diabetes insipidus who cannot produce vasopressin or its neurophysin also lack pro-pressophysin. The structure of bovine pro-pressophysin has now been determined by recombinant DNA techniques.[18]

1.4. Immunocytochemical Approaches

1.4.1. Techniques

Gathering most of the new data obtained in the last decade concerning the vasopressin and oxytocin systems in the brain was made possible by the application of immunocytochemical methods, either by immunofluorescence or immunoperoxidase techniques.[19] Both methods provide similar results at the light microscopic level utilizing the same immunological principles. The immunoenzyme techniques, most commonly employing horseradish peroxidase as the enzyme, have the added advantage of permanent labeling and visible reaction products at the ultrastructural level.[20] In addition to being more sensitive than Gomori stains, they can distinguish vasopressin from oxytocin neurons, and others which may be Gomori-positive or -negative. For peptidergic neurons in general, immunocytochemical methods provide the first available approach to chemical identification of specific pathways.[14,19] Chemical neuroanatomy had its beginnings a decade earlier with the application of Falk fluorescence excitation to map catecholamine systems in the brain.[21] New neuroanatomical pathways now are being described that often do not follow the traditional nuclear groups and fiber projections. It will take some time to understand fully the extent, location, and connections, let alone the physiological roles, of the numerous peptidergic pathways in the brain. For the vasopressin–oxytocin system, the source and connections of the extrahypothalamic pathways remain to be fully defined.

1.4.2. Limitations

Some of the limitations of immunocytochemical tools are discussed here prior to the description of vasopressin and oxytocin systems. False negative and false positive results, as well as the possibility that the source of reactive fibers may be too distant from the perikarya of origin to be directly traced, present some of the problems in interpretation. These are important tools, but they are far from perfect.[19]

1.4.2a. False Negative Results.   Lack of reactivity where it should be present has a number of causes, many of which are now known. They include lack of an adequate antibody or failure of its detection system, loss of the antigen from the tissue during processing, destruction or inactivation of antigenic sites by the fixative used, or concentrations of antigen too low to be visualized. Antisera raised for their high titer and affinity for radioimmunassay are not necessarily good for immunocytochemistry. The reverse is sometimes true in that antisera developed for immunocytochemistry are often inadequate for radioimmunoassay. Furthermore, different antibodies in the same antiserum to the same antigen, possibly reacting at different sites, are likely to be selected by the different methods.[22] One cannot assume, therefore, that characterization of titer, affinity, and specificity using one system applies to another. Antigens are known to be lost from the tissues, particularly during dehydration.[23] This is presently being avoided by reaction of vibratome sections prior to dehydration and embedding.[19] Another approach is to use a fixative that conjugates the peptide to the tissue as in the case of acrolein, which reacts with the histidine in thyrotropin-releasing hormone (TRH).[24] Fixatives can also prevent antibody penetration owing to cross-linking of proteins, for example when glutaraldehyde is used in concentrations most ideal for preservation of membranes for electron microscopic study. Improved penetration can be achieved by application of detergents such as Triton X-100 or Saponin, but they disrupt membranes. The reactivity of the reactive sites of the tissue antigen can be blocked by reaction with formaldehyde, if the antigenic site contains an aromatic amino acid such as tyrosine or phenylalanine.[25] Poor reactivity in perikaryal sites of origin compared to terminals that contain higher concentrations of peptide antigen can be increased by prior administration of colchicine. Colchicine blocks axonal transport and causes a buildup of the peptide in the cell body.

1.4.2b. Specificity.   Given the best absorption controls, the inherent limitation of immunocytochemistry is the inability of the method to distinguish between reactivity with the antigenic determinants of the substance (antigen) in question, or with another, often unknown, substance that shares these determinants.[19] In this regard, immunocytochemistry is not perfect chemistry. Many antisera raised to vasopressin cross-react with oxytocin. If one did not know about oxytocin, which differs in amino acid composition from vasopressin by only two of nine amino acids, application of such an antiserum could lead to the conclusion that all cells in the supraoptic nucleus contain vasopressin, which they do not. There is also the concern that a neuron may take up, but not produce, the stainable substance, as shown recently in the case of albumin.[26] At present, one way around these problems, at least in part, is the demonstration of two or more parts of the precursor or its peptide products in the same neuron by simultaneous or sequential visualization using antibodies to different antigenic determinants. For example the co-localization of vasopressin and its neurophysin in the same neuron[19,27] is stronger evidence that the neuron can produce the substance in question. Even more antigens and corresponding antibodies to the pro-opiocortin system have been available for co-localization studies.[28,29] The availability of different antibodies to different parts of the same molecule would be very useful for the same type of study. For larger peptides this is being accomplished by raising antisera to fragments.[28,29] For smaller peptides the hybridoma technique offers the possibility of several monoclonal antibodies to different determinants of the same molecule.[25] Another useful approach to the problem on the horizon involves *in situ* hybridization with labeled cDNA directed to the cellular nucleic acid code to the precursor in question.[30] This would indicate that the neuron in question has the specific genetic code. Whether it is translated into precursor and products could then be determined by immunocytochemistry.

2. MAGNOCELLULAR VASOPRESSIN AND OXYTOCIN SYSTEMS

2.1. Cells Contributing to the Neurohypophysial Pathway

It is now known through retrograde tracing experiments with dyes or horseradish peroxidase placed in posterior pituitary that all of the magnocellular neurons in the supraoptic nuclei and those in the paraventricular nuclei and accessory groups are the source of the fibers in the hypothalamo-neurohypophysial tract[31-35] (Table I). The supraoptic nucleus contributes many more fibers to the hypothalamo-neurohypophysial tract than does the paraventricular nucleus. The cell bodies in paraventricular nucleus that project to posterior pituitary lie in the medial and lateral magnocellular subnuclei. Some parvocellular (small) neurons in paraventricular nucleus and few if any parvocellular neurons in suprachiasmatic nucleus project to the posterior pituitary.[33,34] Although some of the smaller neurons in paraventricular nucleus also contain oxytocin or vasopressin, most project to extrahypothalamic sites; those containing vasopressin in the medial parvocellular region project to the portal capillary system in the zona externa of the median eminence.[34,36] Many small neurons containing TRH[22] or neurotensin[37] are also found in this region

TABLE I. Neurosecretory Projections Containing Oxytocin or Vasopressin[a]

Terminal field	Origin (nucleus)	Peptide
Posterior pituitary	Magnocellular	
	Paraventricular	
	Anterior	OT
	Medial magnocellular	OT
	Medial and lateral	OT, VP
	Supraoptic	OT, VP
	Accessory	OT, VP
	Circularis	
	Forebrain bundle	
	Bed stria terminalis	
	Preoptic	
	Zona incerta	
	Substantia innominata	
	Parvocellular PVN	
	Some of all five divisions	OT, VP?
Zona externa of	Parvocellular PVN	VP
median eminence	Medial (mainly dorsal part)	
Organum vasculosum	Suprachiasmatic	VP
	Rostral magnocellular	OT, VP

[a] Abbreviations: OT, oxytocin; PVN, paraventricular nucleus; VP, vasopressin.

(medial paraventricular) and they project to zona externa and/or to the posterior pituitary gland. The medial parvocellular portion of the paraventricular nucleus is continuous with the periventricular nucleus, which also contains somatostatin neurons. These project to both zona externa and posterior pituitary.[38] Enkephalin-containing fibers, possibly arising from neurons in the paraventricular nucleus, also project to posterior pituitary.[39] The term *neurohypophysial peptides*, traditionally applied to vasopressin and oxytocin, is no longer accurate, although they are the predominant hormones of the posterior pituitary gland.

2.2. Distribution of Neurons in the Nuclei

The magnocellular neurosecretory system comprises the oxytocin and vasopressin neurons found in both the supraoptic and paraventricular nuclei, which terminate in the posterior pituitary gland.[31–36] These hormones and

FIGURE 1. Color photomicrographs of two coronal vibratome sections of rat hypothalamus, one immunoreacted with a monoclonal antibody to vasopressin (upper right panel; darkfield), and another double-reacted with monoclonal antibodies to vasopressin (blue) and to oxytocin (brown) (other panels; brightfield). The section in the upper right panel reacted for vasopressin was prepared and reacted as previously described.[25] The tissue was fixed with periodate–lysine–formaldehyde and cut at 100 μm on a vibratome. The section was first reacted wtih a mouse monoclonal antibody specific for vasopressin (IIID-7), followed by rabbit anti-mouse immunoglobulin conjugated to peroxidase. Reaction products were generated with diaminobenzidine. Double reactions were carried out on vibratome sections of another rat prepared and treated as described previously, but using a specific monoclonal antibody to oxytocin (Al-28) and diaminobenzidine to generate the brown color, followed by the antibody to vasopressin and 4-Cl-1 naphthol as the substrate for peroxidase to develop the blue color.

Lower left: Both oxytocin (brown) and vasopressin (blue) neurons are found in supraoptic and paraventricular nuclei. 11 × (on the 35-mm frame of 2 × 2).

Lower right: Higher magnification of the supraoptic nucleus, showing that vasopressin neurons are more concentrated in the ventral part of the nucleus at this level. 54 × (on the 35-mm frame of 2 × 2).

Upper left: Higher magnification of the paraventricular nucleus. At this level of the major wing, vasopressin neurons form a central core in the lateral magnocellular group rimmed by oxytocin neurons. 54 × (on the 35-mm frame of 2 × 2).

Upper right: Photomicrograph of another section of the paraventricular nucleus reacted only with monoclonal antibody specific to vasopressin. Note beaded axonal fibers projecting laterally from the cell bodies through and around the fornix. 27 × (on the 35-mm frame of 2 × 2). All photographs reproduced at 260%. [From A. Hou-Yu (unpublished). Photographs by Alfred T. Lamme, FBPA.]

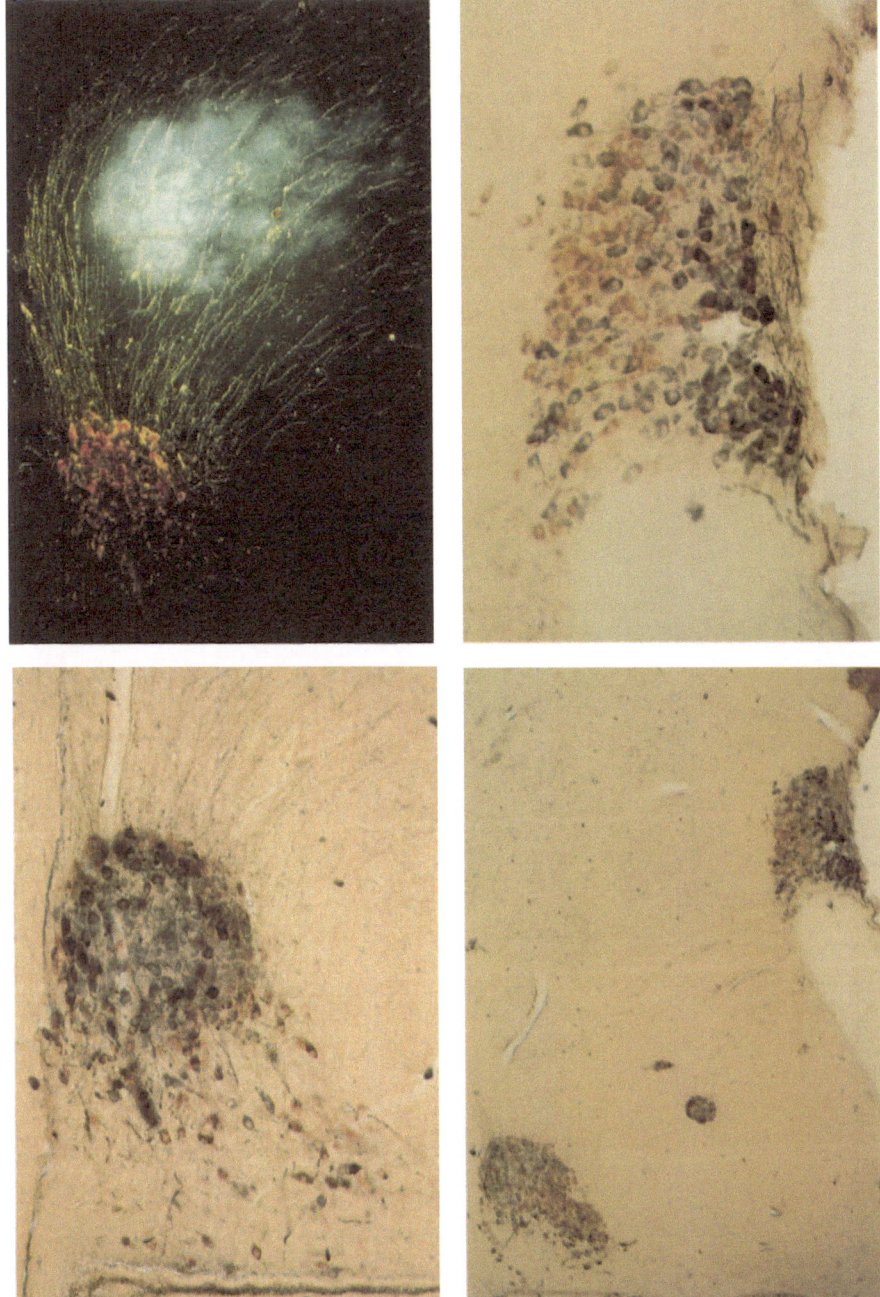

their respective neurophysins are formed in different populations of neurons of the system and are unevenly distributed within the nuclei.[13,20,27,40,41] Oxytocin cells tend to be more concentrated in the rostral parts of each nucleus. The rostral, anterior (commissural) nucleus is solely oxytocin-containing.[42] In the major wing of the paraventricular nucleus (lateral magnocellular) vasopressin neurons form a central core of cells rimmed by oxytocin neurons[20] (Figure 1). At this rostrocaudal level of the hypothalamus, vasopressin cells in the supraoptic nucleus are generally ventral, while oxytocin neurons form a dorsal rim[20,40] (Figure 1). Both types of magnocellular neurons are also found in accessory groups of neurons, which also project to the posterior pituitary (Table I). Some magnocellular neurons are also found near the organum vasculosum of the lamina terminalis (OVLT), where the peptides are found in nerve terminals.[43] This may serve as another neurosecretory pathway for these hormones. As in the case of luteinizing-hormone-releasing hormone and somatostatin neurons that terminate at this site,[14,38] the functions of vasopressin and oxytocin in the OVLT are unknown.

By electrophysiological criteria,[7,8] as well as by immunocytochemical analysis, vasopressin and oxytocin neurons function separately. During suckling, which induces oxytocin release, intracellular recordings reveal a characteristic firing pattern in oxytocinergic neurons in both the supraoptic and paraventricular nuclei. Under these conditions vasopressinergic neurons show no electrophysiological change. On the other hand these cells demonstrate a phasic or bursting pattern during stimulation of vasopressin release. That phasic cells actually contain vasopressin was recently demonstrated in hypothalamo-neurohypophysial explants in which intracellular recording, dye marking, and immunocytochemistry were carried out on the same cells in the rat.[44]

2.3. Course of the Pathway

The main fiber pathway arising from the paraventricular nucleus is made up of axons passing laterally around and through the fornix (Figure 1), which turn ventrally to pass over and join the axons from the supraoptic nucleus to form a tract converging in the zona interna of the median eminence. The pathway then continues down the pituitary stalk to end on basement membranes of the capillaries in the posterior pituitary gland.[20,40,45]

2.4. Other Peptides in the System

Other peptides have been described in magnocellular neurons and may coexist with oxytocin or vasopressin in the same neuron. Cholecystokinin was found in oxytocin neurons[46] and dynorphin in those containing vasopressin.[47] The syntheses of dynorphin and vasopressin are under different genetic controls in the same cell, as shown by the finding that dynorphin persists in these cells, which are present but lack vasopressin Brattleboro rats.[20] On the other hand, angiotensin II immunoreactivity,[48] which is detected in vasopressin neurons, disappears together with vasopressin immunoreactivity in Brattleboro rats (even when hyperactivity of this system is suppressed by chronic vasopressin treatment). This suggests that angiotensin-II-like material is linked to vasopressin biosynthesis. How it is related is uncertain since bovine pro-pressophysin possesses no amino acid sequences in common with angiotensin II. Met-enkephalin and leu-enkephalin have been reported in oxytocin and vasopressin fibers, respectively, and they may actually coexist with the hormones in the same granules.[49] The functional significance of the coexisting peptides in neurohypophysial secretion is not known. Enkephalin is thought to be the opiate that inhibits oxytocin secretion at the pituitary level.[50] Whether this might be accomplished by an intracellular or a preterminal autoreceptor mechanism is not known. Dopamine fibers ending near vasopressin terminals probably act to inhibit vasopressin secretion.[51]

3. PARVOCELLULAR VASOPRESSIN SECRETORY SYSTEM TO MEDIAN EMINENCE

3.1. History of Vasopressin Secretion into Portal Blood

Whether or not vasopressin has a role in anterior pituitary function, particularly in regard to the stimulation of adrenocorticotropic hormone (ACTH) secretion, has long been debated.[52] Although suggested by experiments in the 1950s,[53,54] this possibility was subsequently generally discounted as an important issue for several reasons. The amounts of vasopressin secreted into hypophysial portal blood were estimated to have to reach concentrations of about a thousandfold higher than those found in the peripheral circulation in order to release ACTH.[54] Moreover, there was bioassay evidence that a corticotropin-releasing factor was present in hypothalamic extracts that was more potent than and different from vasopressin.[55–57] Regulation of the pituitary–adrenal axis was found to be only moderately abnormal in the vasopressin-deficient Brattleboro rat.[58] By electron microscopy the granules found in axon terminals in zona externa of the median eminence were smaller (approximately 100 nm diameter) than those known to contain vasopressin in posterior pituitary gland (120–180 nm).[59] Gomori-positive terminals in zona externa whose content of stainable neurosecretory material is increased after adrenalectomy were assumed to contain corticotropin-releasing factor and not vasopressin, because it was the smaller granules that increased in these axons.[60]

3.2. New Evidence for a Vasopressin Pathway to Median Eminence

The first major new finding related to neurohypophysial control of the adenohypophysis that was made when immunocytochemical techniques were employed was the discovery of neurophysin-containing terminals in the zona externa of the median eminence of sheep[61] and monkeys.[62] This was subsequently shown to be predominately a vasopressin rather than an oxytocin terminal region.[63,64] By immunoelectron microscopy, vasopressin and its neurophysin were found to be contained in the smaller granules in nerve terminals near portal capillaries.[46,64] Adrenalectomy was associated with marked increases in vasopressin content in these terminals.[64] Glucocorticoid replacement prevented these increases.[64,65] Vasopressin concentrations in individual portal vein plasma measured by radioimmunoassay were found to be 100–1000 times higher than those in peripheral blood in monkeys[62] and rats.[66,67] These findings reopened the question of a role for the hormone in ACTH regulation. They suggested a direct secretory system into portal blood and an inhibitory feedback loop from the adrenal cortex. See Chapter 5 for further discussion of the role of vasopressin in ACTH regulation.

Source of Fibers to Zona Externa.   At the time of the discovery of zona externa neurophysin-containing fibers a decade ago, it was correctly assumed that they arose from the paraventricular rather than the supraoptic nucleus.[61] It had previously been shown that removal of the posterior pituitary gland or low stalk section was associated with loss of most or all neurons in the supraoptic nucleus and only some of those in the paraventricular nucleus.[68] This can now be explained by the knowledge that all terminals of the supraoptic nucleus end in posterior pituitary, while many more fibers from the paraventricular nucleus terminate on capillaries above such lesions in the upper stalk or median eminence, or even project elsewhere in the brain (Figure 2) and are therefore spared by such lesions. It also explains why permanent or

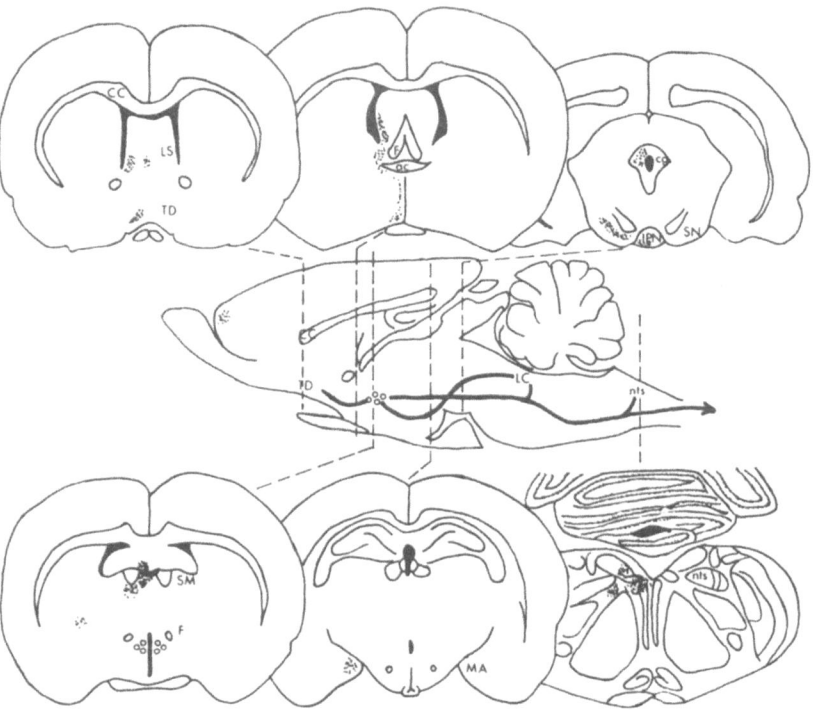

FIGURE 2. Diagrammatic representation of the major extrahypothalamic projections of the vasopressin neurosecretory system in the rat brain. The sagittal illustration depicts the major efferent fiber pathways that appear to originate predominately from the paraventricular nucleus of the hypothalamus (open circles). The major descending projection continues further caudally to the spinal cord (arrow). The drawings of the coronal sections are taken from the various planes depicted (dashed lines) and illustrate the terminal fields of innervation of these extrahypothalamic projections. CC, corpus callosum; F, fornix; IPN, intrapeduncular nucleus; LC, locus ceruleus; LS, lateral septum; MA, medial amygdala; SM, striae medullaris; SN, substantia nigra; TD, tractus diagonalis; ac, anterior commissure; cg, central gray; nts, nucleus tractus solitarius. (Modified from refs. 86 and 91.)

significant diabetes insipidus does not recur after removal of the posterior pituitary gland, as such neurosecretory terminals can take over, perhaps in part by sprouting, to form new connections with blood vessels in the stalk–median eminence.[69,70] What was not appreciated initially was the smaller size and location of the vasopressin neurons in the paraventricular nucleus that contribute to this pathway.[36] The smaller granules in this neurosecretory system are now thought to come primarily from the dorsal part of the medial parvocellular portion of the paraventricular nucleus[33,34,36] (Table I).

3.3. Continuing Controversies

3.3.1. Source of Portal Vein Vasopressin

Whether the large amounts of vasopressin found in hypophysial portal blood are directly secreted by the paraventricular median eminence system or arrive there by retrograde portal flow from the posterior pituitary gland is not totally resolved. A tenfold reduction in portal vein vasopressin content was found after removal of the posterior pituitary gland in one study,[66] and no change was found in another.[67] Support for the importance of the direct pathway to median eminence was obtained by differential electrical stimulation of the paraventricular and supraoptic nuclei in cats.[71] Stimulation of the paraventricular released ACTH and vasopressin into the peripheral circulation, while only vasopressin was released by stimulation of the supraoptic nucleus. However, there was some decline in ACTH with supraoptic stimulation, suggesting the possibility of release of an inhibiting substance and making interpretation of these results less than totally clear.

It is also not yet known whether the increases in zona externa vasopressin content are associated with increased or decreased vasopressin secretion. Direct measurements of portal vein content after adrenalectomy are needed to establish these possibilities. Adrenalectomy has been shown to be associated with selective increases in RNA turnover[72] and vasopressin biosynthesis[73] in the paraventricular–median eminence vasopressin system. Because of this evidence for a specific vasopressin pathway to the portal system, which apparently functions differently from the magnocellular neurosecretory system, our bias at the present is toward the assumption that the large amounts of vasopressin in portal blood primarily comes from the direct system. Ascending catecholamine fibers, mainly noradrenergic, differentially innervate the two secretory systems[74]; their depletion by reserpine causes loss of vasopressin in zona externa, but not in the posterior pituitary.[75]

3.3.2. Vasopressin and Corticotropin-Releasing Factor

Experiments in which antiserum to vasopressin blocked the corticotropin-releasing activity of hypothalamic extracts were interpreted to indicate that vasopressin may be the major corticotropin-releasing factor.[52,76] Other studies had suggested that the function of vasopressin in this regard was to potentiate a different, more potent hypothalamic factor.[52,57,58] These issues will probably be more fully resolved in the near future by comparison of vasopressin with the chemically identified corticotropin-releasing factor recently isolated from ovine hypothalamus.[77] The 41-amino-acid sequence contains neither vasopressin nor sulfur groups that would react with Gomori stains. It is of interest that preliminary immunocytochemical studies indicate that it is also found in neurons of the paraventricular nucleus that project to median eminence. Their relationship to vasopressin neurons, if any, remains to be determined.

3.4. Effects of Glucocorticoids

Glucocorticoids, and not mineralocorticoid replacement, inhibit zona externa increases in vasopressin.[65] It is not known, however, whether this apparent inhibitory feedback of the adrenal cortex acts by a mechanism involving direct effects on the nucleus of the vasopressin cell or indirectly via other steroid-sensitive neurons projecting from elsewhere.

The cause of the relatively long time course required for increases in zona externa vasopressin to take place was recently investigated.[78] There are incremental increases in both content and numbers of fibers visualized beginning at five days and continuing for three to four weeks. Two possible explanations for this phenomenon include sprouting of fiber projections or filling of fibers already present. We have found that the increases with adrenalectomy are not due to sprouting. However, sprouting does occur if a bilateral adrenalectomy is combined with a unilateral lesion of the paraventricular nucleus. Neither adrenalectomy nor unilateral lesioning alone produces this effect. Twenty-six days after the unilateral lesion in a previously adrenalectomized rat, vasopressin fibers grow across the median eminence from the normal side to innervate the denervated zona externa.

4. PARVOCELLULAR SYSTEMS

4.1. Vasopressin in the Suprachiasmatic Nucleus

The second new finding derived from immunocytochemical studies was the discovery that neurophysin and vasopresin immunoreactivity was present in the small cells of the suprachiasmatic nucleus.[14,41,79,80] This was the first suggestion that the hormone could be produced by neurons smaller than magnocellular neurons. Neurophysin as well as vasopressin was absent from these cells in Brattleboro rats, suggesting that these cells produced the vasopressin precursor.[14,80] Oxytocin and its related neurophysin were absent from the suprachiasmatic nucleus, although present in some scattered magnocellular neurons nearby. At the largest part of the nucleus in rats the vasopressin neurons are concentrated in its dorsal and medial parts, although they are present throughout its rostrocaudal extent. Reactive fibers arising from these cells are probably the source of axosomatic vasopressin terminals with other neurons in the nucleus. Neurons containing vasoactive intestinal polypeptide immunoreactivity tend to be concentrated in basal cells of the nucleus[81,82] and also form dense plexuses within it. Ultrastructural studies have shown that axons containing vasoactive intestinal polypeptide form axodendritic synapses within the nucleus.[82] It appears therefore that a major function of these two types of peptidergic neurons in the suprachiasmatic nucleus is to innervate the nucleus itself, which they do by forming dense plexuses. Some fibers also cross to innervate the opposite half of the nucleus.[81]

4.1.1. Projections from the Nucleus

Vasopressin projections also extend out of the suprachiasmatic nucleus to innervate other brain regions.[82–86] Where these fibers terminate is not totally clear as they are hard to separate from those arising from the paraventricular. Some investigators consider the vasopressin fibers to forebrain regions to arise primarily from the suprachiasmatic nucleus[85] while others report its contributions to be more limited to lateral septum and habenula, and midbrain[83] (see Table II). In order to determine the relative contributions of these two nuclei to extrahypothalamic vasopressin projections, additional studies with tracing and lesioning methods will be required.

Neurons containing vasoactive intestinal polypeptide in the suprachias-

TABLE II. Oxytocin, Vasopressin, or Neurophysin in Extrahypothalamic Fibers[a]

Terminal field	Origin	Peptide
Spinal cord		
Lamina I (dorsal horn)	PVN	OT, VP, NP
Lamina X (central gray)	PVN	OT, VP, NP
Intermediolateral gray	PVN	OT, VP, NP
Brainstem		
Substantia nigra	PVN	OT, VP, NP
Mesencephalic gray	SCN	VP
	PVN	OT, NP
Dorsal raphe	SCN	VP
	PVN	OT
Parabrachial	PVN	OT, VP, NP
Locus ceruleus	PVN	NP
Raphe magnus	PVN	OT, VP
Tractus solitarius	PVN	OT, VP, NP
Dorsal motor vagus	PVN	OT, VP, NP
Ambiguus	PVN	OT, VP
Lateral reticular	PVN	OT, VP
Commissural	PVN	OT, VP, NP
Forebrain		
Cortex	PVN	VP, OT, NP
Medial septal	PVN	VP, OT
Lateral septal	SCN, PVN	VP
Diagonal band	SCN, PVN	VP, NP
Amygdala		
Medial	PVN	VP, OT, NP
	SCN	VP
Central, lateral, basal	PVN	VP, OT
Medial-dorsal thalamus	SCN	VP
Lateral habenula	SCN	VP
Dorsal, ventral hippocampus	PVN	VP, OT
Subcommissural organ	SCN	VP

[a] Abbreviations: NP, neurophysin; OT, oxytocin; PVN, paraventricular nucleus; SCN, suprachiasmatic nucleus; VP, vasopressin.

matic nucleus also project to other brain sites, including the paraventricular nucleus where the axons appear to terminate around its ventral border.[81]

4.1.2. Diurnal Rhythms and Vasopressin Secretion

Since the suprachiasmatic nucleus has been implicated in the generation of diurnal rhythms,[81,87] the question arises as to whether vasopressin or vasoactive intestinal polypeptide produced by its neurons have any role in mediating these functions. There is no information available concerning vasoactive intestinal polypeptide in this regard. Vasopressin does not appear to play a critical role since Brattleboro rats deficient in vasopressin have normal drinking and locomotor activity[52] and the expected rhythms in pineal N-acetyltransferase and adrenal cortical function.[81] Recent reports of a diurnal rhythm in vasopressin concentration in cerebrospinal fluid in cats[88] and monkeys[89] not present in the peripheral circulation may suggest that the suprachiasmatic nucleus is the source of independent secretion of the peptide into the ventricular system. However, oxytocin and its neurophysin follow the same rhythm in cerebrospinal fluid.[89] Since they are not present within suprachiasmatic neurons, it seems more likely that other vasopressin and oxytocin pathways are the source of these peptides in cerebrospinal fluid, possibly the paraventricular nucleus. Whether fibers containing these hormones actually penetrate the ependyma and secrete directly into the ventricular system or indirectly by diffusion across the ependyma has been a recent subject of debate among anatomists.[90] Many immunoreactive fibers come close to the ependyma, but it is hard to prove that they actually penetrate it. For functional purposes, the argument is probably not important, since these peptides can freely diffuse into cerebrospinal fluid.

4.2. Extrahypothalamic Systems

4.2.1. A "Hypothalamic Brain Center"

One of the unexpected findings that followed the development of immunohistochemical methods for the study of neurophysin was the demonstration of neurophysin-containing fibers in many regions of the brain and spinal cord that appear to arise from cell bodies in the hypothalamus.[4,36,81,92]

Such pathways from the paraventricular nucleus were suggested by previous anatomical studies using orthograde[93] and retrograde[94] tracing methods. Another neuronal system connected to many of the same brain regions with its center in the hypothalamus is the ACTH/β-endorphin system, which primarily arises in the arcuate nucleus of the hypothalamus.[28,29] A significant difference between the two systems is the relatively scanty projections of the arcuate system to the spinal cord.

4.2.2. Projection Areas

Vasopressin and/or oxytocin have been reported in most of the neurophysin projection areas,[95-99] as reviewed in Table II. Most of the areas listed as terminal fields have been determined by light microscopic criteria in most cases. These need to be confirmed and the type of synapses defined by immunohistochemistry at the ultrastructural level. Axo-dendritic synapses have been demonstrated in habenula and septum that contain vasopressin, and others in medial amygdala that contain oxytocin.[84] Some reactive fibers in some fields could be passing through the region or possibly ending on blood vessels.[100]

4.2.3. Chemical Nature of Extrahypothalamic Hormones

In addition to the limited anatomical data concerning synapses, the biochemical processes and the nature of the peptide products in the extrahypothalamic efferent system remain to be fully defined. In most cases colocalization of vasopressin and oxytocin with their respective neurophysins remains to be studied. Radioimmunoassay of extracts of various regions in rat brain[101,102] indicates the presence of relatively large amounts of vasopressin in forebrain and oxytocin in hindbrain, results that generally support immunocytochemical findings. We have found bioassayable oxytocin in spinal cord (J. D. Haldar, G. Nilaver, and E. A. Zimmerman, unpublished). It has also been recently demonstrated that [^{35}S]cystine incorporated into neurophysin in the paraventricular nucleus is rapidly transported to spinal cord.[103] This is blocked by colchicine administration, as is transport of labeled neurophysins and hormones to the posterior pituitary gland. These findings suggest that the descending system synthesizes and transports neurophysin in a manner similar to the neurosecretory system. Further biochemical characterization of the extrahypothalamic pathways, particularly in regard to vasopressin and oxytocin, is greatly needed, making use of sophisticated chromatographic procedures and radioreceptor techniques.

4.3. Cells of Origin and Trajectory

4.3.1. Rostral Systems

The localization of cells of origin and their contribution to extra hypothalamic regions is complex and as yet not fully resolved, particularly in the case of vasopressin fibers. The supraoptic nucleus does not appear to contribute to these pathways. The suprachiasmatic nucleus or the paraventricular nucleus, or both, may contribute fibers to forebrain and midbrain regions (Table II; Figure 2). Vasopressin projections from the suprachiasmatic nucleus to lateral septum, medial-dorsal thalamus, diagonal band, lateral habenula, medial amygdala, and interpeduncular nucleus, and in midbrain, mesencephalic gray, and dorsal raphe have been proposed.[83,85,86,95] The suprachiasmatic nucleus may also contribute fibers to the organum vasculosum[83,85] and the subcommissural organ.[83] The paraventricular nucleus has also been reported to project to many of the same areas as well as to additional regions, including hippocampus.[4,36,83–85,90–92,95–99] Both vasopressin and oxytocin fibers enter the dorsal and ventral hippocampus, amygdala, and central gray.[83,85] Electrophysiological studies have confirmed direct connections between paraventricular nucleus and lateral septum, amygdala, midbrain, and medulla.[104,105] Scattered fibers containing oxytocin, vasopressin, or neurophysin have been found in the cerebral cortex. Our results suggest that more are found in temporal cortex. Those in entorhinal cortex were reported to arise from the paraventricular nucleus.[83]

4.3.2. Caudal Pathways

4.3.2a. Projections. More extensive studies have been carried out on the descending projections from the paraventricular nucleus to the brainstem and spinal cord.[4,36,83,85,91,92,96–99] Two pathways have been described.[91,92] One travels caudally in the mesencephalic central gray, and the other, larger pathway travels along the medial forebrain bundle into the ventral tegmental area to form a dense band between the medial lemniscus and the zona compacta of the substantia nigra. Although both oxytocin and vasopressin fibers have been reported in substantia nigra, those containing oxytocin appear to predominate.[92] More caudally in the midbrain fibers pass dorsomedially to innervate the parabrachial nuclei and locus ceruleus. The main ventrolateral bundle continues into the pons and medulla and then arches dorsomedially, particularly at the level of the lateral reticular nucleus, which it innervates. Some fibers also enter the nucleus raphe magnus. In the dorsal medulla, the commissural nucleus, solitary tract, and dorsal motor vagal nuclei are heavily innervated. Again, these appear to be predominantly oxytocin fibers, although those containing vasopressin are also present. In this region vasopressin fibers may be more relatively concentrated in the dorsal motor vagal nucleus.[92]

The major caudal pathway continues into the spinal cord in the dorsolateral funiculus. Some fibers also descend in the central gray (lamina X). Both fiber systems travel the entire length of the cord. Innervation patterns are found in the marginal zone of the dorsal horn (lamina I), the central gray (lamina X), and the intermediolateral gray. The spinal cord is more heavily innervated in some regions than in others.[96] In the rat the most dense accumulations of fibers in intermediolateral gray are found at the T1–3, T9–11, and T13–L2 levels.[36,96]

4.3.2b. Cells of Origin.   That these fibers originate in the paraventricular nucleus is suggested by their disappearance after bilateral lesions of the nucleus[92] and by blockade of neurophysin transported from the nucleus by intraventricular injections of colchicine.[103] This was also demonstrated by combined retrograde tracing and immunocytochemical methods in which most of the labeled cells were found to be located in the dorsal, lateral, and ventral aspects of the medial paravocellular divisions of the paraventricular nucleus, although some posterior magnocellular neurons also reacted.[34,36,97,98] Twice as many peptide-identified perikarya in the paraventricular nucleus project to spinal cord than medulla, and the ratio of vasopressin to oxytocin cells was 2:1 for cord and 4:1 for medulla.[36,99] Other transmitterlike substances are expected to be found in the descending pathway, since vasopressin and oxytocin account for only about 10% of the labeled neurons.[36] Somatostatin and dopamine[36] may contribute, as well as neurotensin[37] or TRH,[22] which is found in medial parvocellular neurons in the paraventricular nucleus. Double simultaneous retrograde tracing studies using two different colored dyes, each placed in different target sites, revealed that separate neurons in the para-ventricular nucleus generally project to different regions.[36,97] Only about 15% of the labeled neurons in paraventricular nucleus contained both dyes when one was placed in the medulla and the other in the spinal cord. Similar studies indicated that neurons sending fibers to posterior pituitary or median eminence do not usually project to medulla or spinal cord.[36,97,98]

5. FUNCTIONAL ROLES OF VASOPRESSIN PATHWAYS

5.1. Forebrain Functions

Although incomplete, the data already available suggest multiple new roles for vasopressin in the central nervous system in addition to neurosecre-tory functions in posterior and anterior pituitary gland. Projections to fore-brain, or perhaps others to the ventricular system, may provide the anatomical substrate for vasopressin enhancement of memory and alertness.[106,107] Fibers to the lateral septum and/or amygdala may inhibit fever responses to pyro-gens.[108]

5.2. Autonomic Control

Connections with neurons of the sympathetic and parasympathetic system in brainstem and spinal cord suggest additional roles for vasopressin as well as oxytocin in the central regulation of autonomic function.[36,74] It has been postulated that vasopressin projections to locus ceruleus may modify the changes in brain capillary permeability, controlled by norepinephrine fibers originating from this nucleus, which responds in turn to changes in plasma osmolality and blood pressure.[109]

5.2.1. Interaction with the Parasympathetic System

Several interesting possibilities for autonomic interaction arise in regard to the efferent projections from the paraventricular nucleus to the parasym-pathetic neurons of the medulla. The nucleus of the solitary tract receives visceral sensory information from cranial nerves IX and X concerning blood pressure and volume and relays it to the hypothalamus to regulate vasopressin secretion.[36] Similarly, hemodynamic changes that release ACTH are relayed via the dorsal motor vagus as well as the nucleus of the solitary tract.[110] The descending vasopressin system could modulate its own secretion as well as that of ACTH by its projections to these nuclei. Since these connections are reciprocal, the ascending connections to the paraventricular nucleus may, in turn, selectively affect or differentially regulate the neurosecretory and possibly the descending efferent vasopressin neurons. The possibility of a very sophisticated and selective servomechanism in this regard is further suggested by different norepinephrine projections to the paraventricular nucleus: Those to parvocellular neurons arise from the solitarius region, while innervation of magnocellular portions originates from the lateral reticular region.[74] The latter nucleus is, in turn, innervated by the solitarius. It remains to be determined whether a particular vasopressin neuron in the paraventricular nucleus projects to the same brainstem relay neuron that projects to it, and the possible other connections it may have with neurosecretory sites or other neurons are still unclear. The descending connections with the solitary and vagal nuclei may also have a role in the regulation of heart rate and blood pressure.[36]

5.2.2. Sympathetic System

Projections to the preganglionic sympathetic neurons in spinal cord suggest roles for vasopressin in regulating peripheral sympathetic tone. It may be functionally significant that the T9–11 intermediolateral gray neurons innervate kidney and adrenal glands.[36] The central vasopressin system to these neurons may thereby regulate blood flow to these regions, which in turn are known to influence vasopressin secretory pathways via changes in osmolality or glucocorticoid secretion. Fiber pathways to the dorsal horn of the spinal cord or midbrain central gray may account for the analgesic effects of vasopressin.[111]

5.3. Coordination of Stress Responses?

The full extent and nature of the anatomical substrate of vasopressin systems of the brain remain to be defined. Given the newness and incompleteness of this information, it is not surprising that our understanding of its physiological meaning is only fragmentary at this time. A simplified traditional functional concept for such a widespread vasopressin system originating from a central station in the hypothalamus may involve coordination of different but related functions in response to stress: vasopressin and adrenal responses by the neurosecretory systems, activation of alertness and memory by forebrain pathways, blood pressure and heart rate by brainstem connections, and analgesia by projections to midbrain central gray or spinal cord. These possibilities do not preclude other functions for vasopressin as well. For example, it is difficult to incorporate the possible physiological role of the slow diurnal changes in cerebrospinal fluid vasopressin[88] concentrations into a rapid stress-related mechanism.

6. ADDENDUM

The coexistence of vasopressin with corticotropin-releasing factor in parvocellular neurons in the medial paraventricular nucleus has now been demonstrated by several laboratories.[112–114]

ACKNOWLEDGMENTS. The authors thank Dr. Susan Rosario and Ann Sollas for technical assistance; Alfred T. Lamme, FBPA, for color photography; and Anna Silberstein for help with the manuscript.

Work reported herein was supported by USPHS Grants AM 20337 and HD 13147.

REFERENCES

1. Scharrer E, Scharrer B: Hormones produced in neurosecretory cells. *Rec Prog Horm Res* 10:183–240, 1954.
2. Sloper JC: The experimental and cytopathological investigation of neurosecretion in the hypothalamus and pituitary, in Harris GW, Donovan BT (eds): *The Pituitary Gland*. Berkeley, University of California Press, 1966, vol 3, p 131.
3. Scharrer E, Scharrer B: Secretory cells within the hypothalamus. *Res Publ Assoc Nerv Ment Dis* 20:170–194, 1940.
4. Zimmerman EA: The organization of oxytocin and vasopressin pathways, in Martin JB, Reichlin S, Bick KL (eds): *Neurosecretion and Brain Peptides*. New York, Raven Press, 1981, p 63.
5. Sachs H, Fawcett P, Takabatake Y, et al: Biosynthesis and release of vasopressin and neurophysin. *Rec Prog Horm Res* 25:447–484, 1969.

6. Brownstein MJ, Russell JT, Gainer H: Synthesis, transport and release of posterior pituitary hormones. *Science* 207:373–378, 1980.

7. Cross BA, Dyball RE, Dyer RG, et al: Endocrine neurones. *Rec Prog Horm Res* 31:243–294, 1975.

8. Poulain DA, Wakerley JB: Electrophysiology of hypothalamic magnocellular neurones secreting oxytocin and vasopressin. *Neuroscience* 7:773–808, 1982.

9. Gomori G: Observations with differential stains on human islets of Langerhans. *Am J Pathol* 17:395–406, 1941.

10. Du Vigneaud V: Hormones of the posterior pituitary gland: Oxytocin and vasopressin. *Harvey Lect* 1954–1955:1–26, 1956.

11. Bargmann W, Scharrer E: The site of origin of the hormones of the posterior pituitary. *Am Sci* 39:255–259, 1951.

12. Barry PG: Les voies neurosécrétoires extra-hypophysaires et le problème de l'action nerveuse centrale des hormones posthypophysaires. *Le Jour Med Lyon* 20:1065–1074, 1958.

13. Vandesande F, Dierickx K: Identification of vasopressin-producing and/or oxytocin-producing neurons in the hypothalamic magnocellular neurosecretory system of the rat. *Cell Tissue Res* 164:153–162, 1975.

14. Zimmerman EA: Localization of hypothalamic hormones by immunocytochemical techniques, in Martini L, Ganong WF (eds): *Frontiers in Neuroendocrinology*. New York, Raven Press, 1976, vol 4, p 25.

15. Olivecrona H: Paraventricular nucleus and pituitary gland. *Acta Physiol Scand* 40(suppl 136):1–178, 1957.

16. Douglas WW: Mechanism of release of neurohypophysial hormones: Stimulus secretion coupling, in Knobil E, Sawyer WH (eds): *Handbook of Physiology, Section 7: Endocrinology*. Washington, DC, American Physiological Society, 1974, p 191.

17. Sachs H, Takabatake Y: Evidence for a precursor in vasopressin biosynthesis. *Endocrinology* 75:943–950, 1964.

18. Land H, Schutz G, Schmale H, et al: Nucleotide sequence of cloned CDNA encoding bovine arginine vasopressin–neurophysin II precursor. *Nature* 295:299–303, 1982.

19. Zimmerman EA, Krupp L, Hoffman DL, et al: Exploration of peptidergic pathways in brain by immunocytochemistry: A ten year perspective. *Peptides* 1(suppl 1):3–10, 1980.

20. Sternberger LA: *Immunocytochemistry*. Englewood Cliffs, New Jersey, Prentice-Hall, 1974.

21. Fuxe K: Evidence for the existence of monoamine neurons in the central nervous system. IV. The distribution of monoamine terminals in the central nervous system. *Acta Physiol Scand* 64(suppl 247):37–85, 1965.

22. Sokol HW, Zimmerman EA, Sawyer WH, et al: The hypothalamo-neurohypophysial system of the rat: Localization and quantification of neurophysin by light microscopic immunocytochemistry in normal rat and in Brattleboro rats deficient in vasopressin and a neurophysin. *Endocrinology* 98:1176–1188, 1976.

23. Goldsmith PC, Ganong WF: Ultrastructural localication of luteinizing hormone-releasing hormone in the median eminence of the rat. *Brain Res* 97:181–193, 1975.

24. Lechan RM, Jackson IMD: Immunohistochemical localization of thyrotropin-releasing hormone in the rat hypothalamus and pituitary. *Endocrinology* 111:55–65, 1982.

25. Hou-Yu A, Ehrlich P, Valiquette G, et al: A monoclonal antibody to vasopressin: Preparation, characterization and application in immunocytochemistry. *J Histochem Cytochem* 30:1249–1260, 1982.

26. Nilaver G, Brem H, Zimmerman EA: Immunocytochemical localization of albumin in rat brain. *Neurology* 32:A107, 1982.

27. Vandesande F, Dierickx K, DeMey J: Identification of the vasopressin–neurophysin II and the oxytocin–neurophysin I producing neurons in the bovine hypothalamus. *Cell Tissue Res* 156:189–200, 1975.

28. Watson SJ, Akil H, Walker JM: Anatomical and biochemical studies of the opioid peptides and related substances in the brain. *Peptides* I(suppl 1):11–20, 1980.
29. Krieger DT, Liotta AS, Brownstein MJ, et al: ACTH, β-lipotropin and related peptides in brain, pituitary and blood. *Rec Prog Horm Res* 36:277–344, 1980.
30. Roberts J, Chen C, Eberwine J, et al: Glucocorticoid regulation of proopiomelanocortin gene expression in rodent pituitary. *Rec Prog Horm Res* 38:227–249, 1982.
31. Sherlock DA, Field PM, Raisman G: Retrograde transport of horseradish peroxidase in the magnocellular neurosecretory system of the rat. *Brain Res* 88:403–414, 1975.
32. Kelly J, Swanson LW: Additional forebrain regions projecting to the posterior pituitary: Preoptic region, bed nucleus of the stria terminalis and zona incerta. *Brain Res* 197:1, 1980.
33. Wiegand SJ, Price JL: Cells of origin of the afferent fibers to the median eminence in the rat. *J Comp Neurol* 192:1–19, 1980.
34. Armstrong WE, Warach S, Hatton GI, et al: Subnuclei in the rat hypothalamic paraventricular nucleus: A cytoarchitectonic, HRP and immunocytochemical analysis. *Neuroscience* 5:1931–1958, 1980.
35. Armstrong WE, Hatton GI: The localization of projection neurons in the rat hypothalamic paraventricular nucleus following vascular and neurohypophysial injections of HRP. *Brain Res Bull* 5:473–477, 1980.
36. Swanson LW, Sawchenko PE: Paraventricular nucleus: A site for the integration of neuroendocrine and autonomic mechanisms. *Neuroendocrinology* 31:410–417, 1980.
37. Kahn D, Abrams GM, Zimmerman EA, et al: Neurotensin neurons in the rat hypothalamus: An immunocytochemical study. *Endocrinology* 107:47–54, 1980.
38. Hökfelt T, Elde R, Fuxe K, et al: Aminergic and peptidergic pathways in the nervous system with special reference to the hypothalamus, in Reichlin S, Baldessarini RJ, Martin JB (eds): *The Hypothalamus*, New York, Raven Press, 1978, p 69.
39. Rossier J, Battenberg E, Pittman Q, et al: Hypothalamic enkephalin neurons may regulate the neurohypophysis. *Nature* 227:653–654, 1979.
40. Defendini R, Zimmerman EA: The magnocellular neurosecretory system of the mammalian hypothalamus, in Reichlin S, Baldessarini RJ, Martin JB (eds): *The Hypothalamus*, New York, Raven Press, 1978, p 137.
41. Swaab DF, Pool CW, Nijveldt F: Immunofluorescence of vasopressin and oxytocin in the rat hypothalamo-neurohypophysial system. *J Neural Transm* 36:195–215, 1975.
42. Rhodes CH, Morrell JI, Pfaff DW: Immunohistochemical analysis of magnocellular elements in rat hypothalamus: Distribution and numbers of neurophysin, oxytocin and vasopressin containing cells. *J Comp Neruol* 198:45–85, 1981.
43. Antunes JL, Zimmerman EA: The hypothalamic magnocellular system of the rhesus monkey: An immunocytochemical study. *J Comp Neurol* 181:539–566, 1978.
44. Reaves TA, Hou-Yu A, Zimmerman EA, et al: Vasopressin neurons in rat supraoptic nucleus: Antidromic identification, lucifer yellow injection and immunocytochemical identification in the hypothalamo-neurohypophysial explant. Abstract, Fall Meeting of the American Physiological Society, 1982.
45. Silverman AJ, Zimmerman EA: Ultrastructural localization of neurophysin and vasopressin in the median eminence and posterior pituitary of the guinea pig. *Cell Tissue Res* 159:291–310, 1975.
46. Vanderhaeghen JJ, Lotstra F, Vandesande F, et al: Coexistance of cholecystokinin and oxytocin–neurophysin in some magnocellular hypothalamo-hypophyseal neurons. *Cell Tissue Res* 221:227–231, 1981.
47. Watson SJ, Akil H, Fischli W, et al: Dynorphin and vasopressin: Common localization in magnocellular neurons. *Science* 216:85–87, 1982.

48. Hoffman DL, Krupp L, Schrag D, et al: Angiotensin immunoreactivity in vasopressin cells in rat hypothalamus and its relative deficiency in homozygous brattleboro rats. *Ann NY Acad Sci* 394:135–141, 1982.

49. Martin R, Voight KL: Enkephalins co-exist with oxytocin and vasopressin in nerve terminals of rat neurohypophysis. *Nature* 289:502–503, 1981.

50. Clarke G, Wood P, Merrick L, et al: Opiate inhibition of peptide release from the neurohumoral terminals of the hypothalamic neurons. *Nature* 282:746–748, 1979.

51. Lightman LS, Iversen LL, Forshing ML: Dopamine and (D-Ala⁶,D-Leu⁵) enkephalin inhibit the electrically stimulated neurohypophyseal release of vasopressin *in vitro:* Evidence for calcium-dependent opiate action. *J Neurosci* 2:78–81, 1982.

52. Gillies G, Lowry PJ: Corticotropin releasing hormone and its vasopressin component, in Ganong WF, Martini L (eds): *Frontiers in Neuroendocrinology*. New York, Raven Press, 1982, vol 7, p 45.

53. McCann SM, Brobeck JR: Evidence for a role of the supraopticohypophysial system in the regulation of adrenocorticotropin secretion. *Proc Soc Exp Biol Med* 87:318–324, 1954.

54. McCann SM: The ACTH releasing activity of extracts of the posterior lobe of the pituitary *in vivo. Endocrinology* 60:664–676, 1957.

55. Schally AV, Arimura A, Kastin AJ: Hypothalamic regulatory hormones. *Science* 179:341–350, 1973.

56. Blackwell RE, Guillemin R: Hypothalamic control of adenohypophysial secretions. *Annu Rev Physiol* 35:357–390, 1973.

57. Krieger DT, Zimmerman EA: The nature of CRF and its relationship to vasopressin, in Martini L, Besser GM (eds): *Clinical Neuroendocrinology*. New York, Academic Press, 1977, p 363.

58. Yates FE, Russell SM, Dallman MF, et al: Potentiation by vasopressin of corticotropin release induced by corticotropin releasing factor. *Endocrinology* 88:3–15, 1971.

59. Knigge KM, Scott DE: Structure and function of the median eminence. *Am J Anat* 129:223–228, 1970.

60. Wittowski W, Bock R: Electron microscopical studies of the median eminence following interference with the feedback system anterior pituitary–adrenal cortex, in Knigge KM, Scott DE, Weindl A (eds): *Brain Endocrine Interaction: Median Eminence Structure and Function*. Basel, Karger, 1972, p 171.

61. Parry HB, Livett BG: A new hypothalamic pathway to the median eminence containing neurophysin and its hypertrophy in sheep with natural Scrapie. *Nature* 242:63–65, 1973.

62. Zimmerman EA, Carmel PW, Husain MK, et al: Vasopressin and neurophysin: High concentrations in monkey hypophyseal portal blood. *Science* 198:925–927, 1973.

63. Vandesande F, Dierickx K, DeMay J: The origin of the vasopressinergic and oxytocinergic fibers of the external region of the median eminence of the rat hypophysis. *Cell Tissue Res* 180:443–452, 1977.

64. Zimmerman EA, Stillman MA, Recht LD, et al: Vasopressin and corticotropin-releasing factor (CRF): An axonal pathway to portal capillaries in the zona externa of the median eminence containing vasopressin and its interaction with adrenal corticoids. *Ann NY Acad Sci* 297:405–419, 1977.

65. Silverman AJ, Hoffman DL, Gadde C, et al: Adrenal steroid inhibition of the vasopressin–neurophysin neurosecretory system to the median eminence of the rat: Differential effects of corticosterone and deosycorticosterone administration after adrenalectomy. *Neuroendocrinology* 32:129–133, 1981.

66. Oliver C, Michal RS, Porter JC: Hypothalamic–pituitary vasculature: Evidence for retrograde flow in pituitary stalk. *Endocrinology* 101:598–604, 1977.

67. Recht LD, Hoffman DL, Haldar J, et al: Vasopressin concentrations in hypophysial portal plasma: Insignificant reduction following removal of the posterior pituitary gland. *Neuroendocrinology* 33:88–90, 1981.
68. Rasmussen AT: Effects of hypophysectomy and hypophysial stalk section on the hypothalamic nuclei of animals and man. *Res Publ Assoc Res Nerv Ment Dis* 20:245–269, 1940.
69. Rothballer AB, Skaryna SC: Morphological effects of pituitary stalk section in the dog, with particular reference to neurosecretory material. *Anat Rec* 136:5–25, 1960.
70. Antunes JL, Crmel PW, Zimmerman EA, et al: Regeneration of the magnocellular system of the rhesus monkey following hypothalamic lesions. *Ann Neurol* 5:462–469, 1979.
71. Dornhorst A, Carlson D, Seif SM, et al: Control of adrenocorticotropin and vasopressin by supraoptic and paraventricular nuclei. *Endocrinology* 108:1420–1424, 1981.
72. Silverman AJ, Gadde CA, Zimmerman EA: The effect of adrenalectomy on the incorporation of ^{3}H-cytidine into RNA in neurophysin and vasopressin positive neurons in the rat hypothalamus. *Neuroendocrinology* 30:285–290, 1980.
73. Russell JT, Brownstein MJ, Gainer H: ^{35}S-cysteine labeled peptides transported to the neurohypophysis of adrenalectomized, lactating and Brattleboro rats. *Brain Res* 201:227–234, 1980.
74. Sawchenko PE, Swanson LW: Central noradrenergic pathways for the integration of hypothalamic neuroendocrine and automatic responses. *Science* 214:685–687, 1981.
75. Seybold V, Elde R, Hökfelt T: Terminals of reserpine-sensitive vasopressin neurophysin neurons in the external layer of the rat median eminence. *Endocrinology* 108:1803–1809, 1981.
76. Gillies G, Lowry PJ: Corticotropin releasing factor may be modulated vasopressin. *Nature* 287:463–464, 1979.
77. Vale W, Spiess J, Rivier C, et al: Characteristics of a 41-residue ovine hypothalamic peptide that stimulates the secretion of corticotropin and β-endorphin. *Science* 213:1394–1397, 1981.
78. Silverman A-J, Zimmerman EA: Adrenalectomy increases sprouting in a peptidergic neurosecretory system. *Neuroscience* 7:2705–2714, 1982.
79. Sofroniew MV, Weindl A: Identification of parvocellular vasopressin neurons in the suprachiasmatic nucleus of a variety of mammals including primates. *J Comp Neurol* 193:659–675, 1980.
80. Swaab DF, Pool CW: Specificity of oxytocin and vasopressin immunofluorescence. *J Endocrinol* 66:263–272, 1975.
81. Card JP, Brecha N, Karten HJ, et al: Immunocytochemical localization of vasoactive intestinal polypeptide-containing cells and processes in the suprachiasmatic nucleus of the rat: Light and electron microscopic analysis. *J Neurosci* 1:1289–1303, 1981.
82. Sims K, Hoffman DL, Said SI, et al: Vasoactive intestinal polypeptide (VIP) in mouse and rat brain: An immunocytochemical study. *Brain Res* 186:165–183, 1980.
83. Buijs RM: Intra- and extrahypothalamic vasopressin and oxytocin pathways in the rat. *Cell Tissue Res* 192:423–435, 1978.
84. Bujis RM, Swaab DF: Immuno-electron microscopic demonstration of vasopressin and oxytocin synapses in the limbic system of the rat. *Cell Tissue Res* 204:355–365, 1979.
85. Sofroniew MV: Projections from vasopressin, oxytocin and neurophysin neurons to neural targets in the rat and human. *J Histochem Cytochem* 28:475–478, 1980.
86. Sofroniew MV, Weindl A: Projections from the parvocellular vasopressin and neurophysin containing neurons of the suprachiasmatic nucleus. *Am J Anat* 153:391–430, 1978.
87. Moore RY, Eichler VB: Loss of a circadian adrenal corticosterone rhythm following suprachiasmatic lesions in the rat. *Brain Res* 42:201–206, 1972.

88. Reppert SM, Artman A, Swaminathan S, et al: Vasopressin exhibits a daily pattern in cerebrospinal fluid but not in blood. *Science* 213:1256–1257, 1981.

89. Perlow MJ, Reppert SM, Artman HA, et al: Oxytocin, vasopressin, and estrogen-stimulated neurophysin: Daily patterns of concentration in cerebrospinal fluid, *Science* 216:1416–1418, 1982.

90. Krisch B: Immunocytochemistry of neuroendocrine systems. *Prog Histochem Cytochem* 13:1–163, 1980.

91. Swanson LW: Immunohistochemical evidence for a neurophysin-containing autonomic pathway arising in the paraventricular nucleus of the hypothalamus. *Brain Res* 128:346–353, 1977.

92. Nilaver G, Zimmerman EA, Wilkins J, et al: Magnocellular hypothalamic projections to the lower brainstem and spinal cord of the rat: Immunocytochemical evidence for the predominance of oxytocin–neurophysin system compared to a vasopressin–neurophysin system. *Neuroendocrinology* 30:150–158, 1980.

93. Conrad LC, Pfaff DW: Efferents from medial basal forebrain and hypothalamus in the rat. II. An autoradiographic study of the anterior hypothalamus. *J Comp Neurol* 169:221–262, 1976.

94. Kuypers HGJM, Maisky VA: Retrograde axonal transport of horseradish peroxidase from spinal cord to brain stem cell groups in the rat. *Neurosci Lett* 1:9–15, 1975.

95. Buijs RM, Swaab DF, Dogeerom J, et al: Intra- and extrahypothalamic vasopressin and oxytocin pathways in the rat. *Cell Tissue Res* 186:423–433, 1978.

96. Swanson LW, McKellar S: The distribution of oxytocin and vasopressin-stained fibers in the spinal cord of the rat and monkey. *J Comp Neurol* 188:87–106, 1979.

97. Swanson LW, Kuypers HGJM: The paraventricular nucleus: Cytoarchitectonic subdivisions and organization of projections to the pituitary, dorsal vagal complex, and spinal cord as demonstrated by retrograde fluorescence double labeling methods. *J Comp Neurol* 194:555–570, 1980.

98. Swanson LW, Sawchenko PE, Wiegand SJ, et al: Separate neurons in the paraventricular nucleus project to the median eminence and to the medulla and spinal cord. *Brain Res* 198:190–195, 1980.

99. Sofroniew MV, Schrell U: Evidence for a direct projection from oxytocin and vasopressin neurons in the hypothalamic paraventricular nucleus to the medulla oblongata: Immuno-histochemical visualization of both the horseradish peroxidase transport and the peptide produced by the same neurons. *Neurosci Lett* 22:211–217, 1981.

100. Recht LD, Nilaver G, Abrams GM, et al: Oxytocin innervation of cerebral blood vessels: A possible role in local vasoregulation. *Neurology* 32:A110, 1982.

101. Dogterom F, Snigdewint FGM, Buijs RM: The distribution of vasopressin and oxytocin in the rat brain. *Neurosci Lett* 9:341–346, 1978.

102. Rossor MN, Iversen LL, Hawthorn J, et al: Extrahypothalamic vasopressin in human brain. *Brain Res* 214:349–355, 1981.

103. Zimmerman EA, Brownstein MJ, Gainer H: Biosynthesis and transport of neurophysins from hypothalamus to spinal cord. *Neurology* 32:A107, 1982.

104. Pittman QJ, Blume HW, Renaud LP: Connections of the hypothalamic paraventricular nucleus with the neurohypophysis, median eminence, amygdala, lateral septum and mid-brain periaqueductal grey. *Brain Res* 215:15–28, 1981.

105. Zerihun L, Harris M: Electrophysiological identification of neurons of paraventricular nucleus sending axons to both the neurohypophysis and the medulla in the rat. *Neurosci Lett* 23:157–160, 1981.

106. Koob GF, LeMoal M, Faffori O, et al: Arginine vasopressin and vasopressin antagonist peptide: Opposite effects on extinction of active avoidance in rats. *Regulatory Peptides* 2:153–163, 1981.
107. Weingartner H, Gold P, Ballenger JC, et al: Effects of vasopressin on human memory functions. *Science* 211:601–603, 1981.
108. Merker G, Blahser S, Zeisberger E: Reactivity pattern of vasopressin-containing neurons and its relation to the antipyretic reaction in the pregnant guinea pig. *Cell Tissue Res* 212:47–61, 1980.
109. Swanson LW, Hartman BK: Biochemical specificity in central pathways related to peripheral and intracerebral homeostatic functions. *Neurosci Lett* 16:55–60, 1980.
110. Ward DG, Gann DS: Inhibitory and facilitatory areas of the dorsal medulla mediting ACTH release in the cat. *Endocrinology* 99:1213–1219, 1976.
111. Bodnar RJ, Zimmerman EA, Nilaver G, et al: Dissociation of cold-water swim and morphine analgesia in Brattleboro rats with diabetes insipidus. *Life Sci* 26:1581–1590, 1980.
112. Tramu G, Croix C, Pillez A: Ability of the CRF immunoreactive neurons of the paraventricular nucleus to produce a vasopressin-like material. Immunohistochemical demonstration in adrenalectomized guinea pigs and rats. *Neuroendocrinology* 37:467–469, 1983.
113. Kiss JZ, Mezey E, Skirboll L: Corticotropin releasing factor (CRF)-immunoreactive neurons of the paraventricular nucleus become vasopressin positive following adrenalectomy. *Proc Natl Acad Sci USA* (in press).
114. Sawchenko P, Swanson LW, Vale WW: Co-expression of CRF- and vasopressin-immunoreactivity in parvocellular neurosecretory neurons of the adrenalectomized rat. *Proc Natl Acad Sci USA* (in press).

3

BIOSYNTHESIS OF VASOPRESSIN AND NEUROPHYSIN

Harold Gainer

1. INTRODUCTION

The present state of information about the biosynthesis of vasopressin and neurophysin stands as a tribute to the prescience of Howard Sachs and his colleagues. These investigators proposed not only that vasopressin was synthesized by the magnocellular neurons in the hypothalmus as a prohormone,[1,2] but also that this prohormone was a common precursor that contained both vasopressin and neurophysin.[3,4] Twenty years after this first proposal of a vasopressin prohormone, an extensive body of data has been accumulated in favor of this hypothesis, and the full sequence of this precursor has recently been elucidated by recombinant DNA techniques.[5]

Many other proteins and peptides, over the intervening years, have been shown to be derived from the posttranslational processing of larger precursor molecules.[6–8] Much has been learned about the cell biological organization of precursor synthesis and processing, and modern criteria for the identification of putative precursors (or prohormones) have been established. These criteria include;

1. Demonstration in classical pulse–chase experiments in intact cellular systems (in vivo or in situ) that a larger form of the peptide is first synthesized and subsequently decreases in radioactivity as the radioactive peptide is formed. Chemical identity between putative precursor and products is usually established in such experiments by immunoprecipitation and peptide mapping procedures.

Harold Gainer • Section on Functional Neurochemistry, Laboratory of Neurochemistry and Neuroimmunology, National Institute of Child Health and Human Development, National Institutes of Health, Bethesda, Maryland 20205.

2. Demonstration by in vitro (cell-free) translation experiments [i.e., mRNA is purified from the synthesizing tissue and incubated in the presence of heterologous cell-free translation systems (e.g., wheat germ and reticulocyte lysates)] that a larger precursor form of the peptide is synthesized. These experiments can also provide information about the signal sequence of the prohormone, and when they are performed in the presence of microsomal membranes it is possible to demonstrate several posttranslational processes (e.g., signal sequence cleavage, glycosylation).

3. Utilization of modern recombinant DNA techniques to clone cDNA obtained from a purified mRNA template using reverse transcriptase. The cloned cDNA can be rapidly sequenced, and from the nucleotide sequence of the precursor (i.e., pre-prohormone) can be deduced.

All these criteria have been fulfilled in the case of the vasopressin precursor. A brief description of some of these studies is now presented.

2. IDENTIFICATION OF THE VASOPRESSIN PRECURSOR

2.1. Studies on Intact Systems (in Vivo)

Early pulse–chase experiments[9,10] were suggestive of the existence of a precursor for vasopressin and neurophysin. These experiments, however, did not contain sufficient biochemical characterization of the newly synthesized polypeptides to establish a convincing case for a putative precursor of either vasopressin or neurophysin. In 1977, our laboratory reported evidence for an approximately 20,000-molecular-weight form of rat neurophysin that behaved like a precursor in pulse–chase experiments in vivo.[11–14] In these experiments, [^{35}S]cysteine was bilaterally injected using stereotactic techniques over the supraoptic nuclei (SONs) of rats. At various times after the injections, the rats were killed, their brains were removed and rapidly frozen, and their SONs were removed by micropunch dissection for analysis.[11] This selective microdissection procedure increased the "signal-to-noise" ratio in these "pulse–chase" studies in order to allow for resolution of the putative precursors and neurophysin products by solely polyacrylamide gel protein separation techniques. Combined with immunoprecipitation studies using antibodies directed against rat neurophysin,[12–14] this approach allowed for the identification of precursors of rat neurophysin.

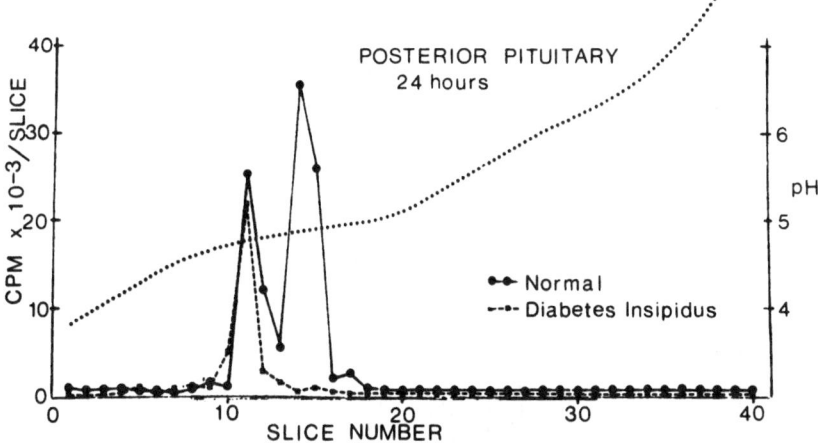

FIGURE 1. Isoelectric focusing (pH 4–6 range ampholytes) of proteins extracted from the posterior pituitaries of normal (solid line) and Brattleboro (broken line) rats 24 hr after injecting [^{35}S]cysteine into the SON. The Brattleboro rats have only one of the two labeled neurophysins (pI 4.6). (From ref. 13.)

The use of the Brattleboro rat (hereditary diabetes insipidus) model in biosynthesis and axonal transport studies, pioneered by Pickering and his colleagues,[15] was instrumental in determining which putative precursor was related to vasopressin.[12–14] Only the oxytocin-associated neurophysin is synthesized and transported to the neural lobe in homozygous Brattleboro rats (for review see ref. 15). Figure 1 illustrates this point by showing that both vasopressin-associated (pI = 4.8) and oxytocin-associated (pI = 4.6) neurophysins are transported to the posterior pituitary in normal rats, but that only the pI 4.6 neurophysin is synthesized and transported in Brattleboro rats. Pulse–chase studies in the SON revealed that at least four larger forms of neurophysin could be resolved by isoelectric focusing.[12–14] At short times after the pulse with [^{35}S]cysteine, two major forms were seen with isoelectric points (pI) of 5.4 and 6.1, followed later by forms with pI values of 5.1 and 5.6 (Figure 2). All four forms were immunoprecipitated by antibodies to rat neurophysin (Figure 3), and only the pI 5.1 and 5.4 forms of the neurophysin precursor were found synthesized in the SONs of Brattelboro rats. Based on these data, we proposed that the pI 6.1 and 5.6 forms were the biosynthetic precursor and intermediate molecular forms, respectively, of the vasopressin-associated neurophysin.[11–14]

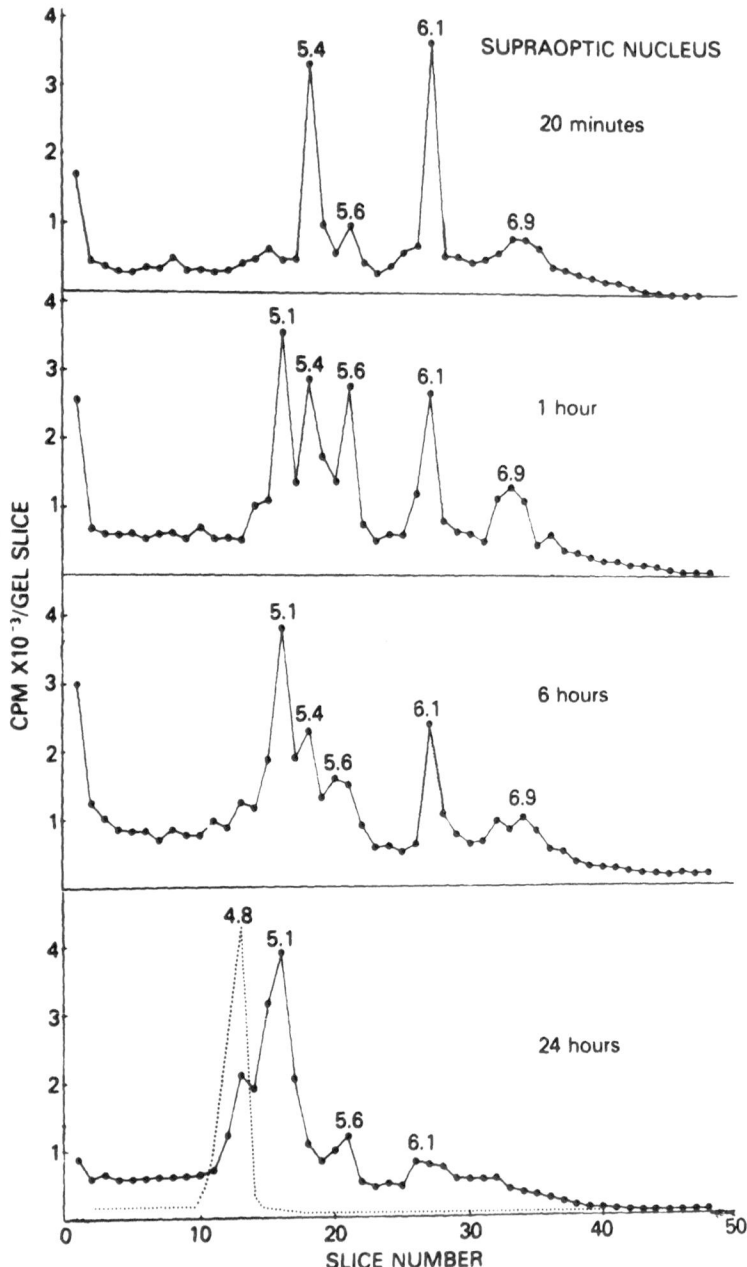

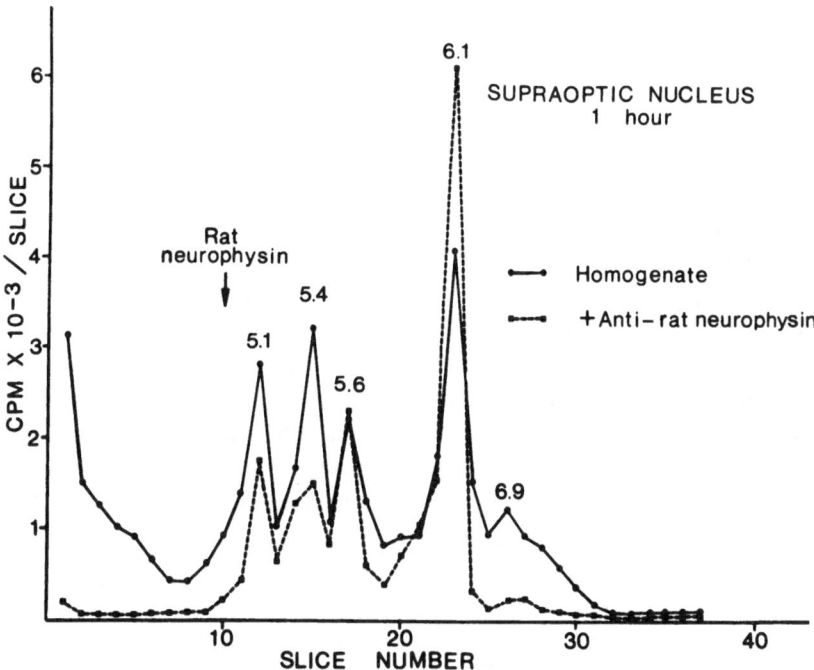

FIGURE 3. Isoelectric focusing of ^{35}S-labeled proteins in an acid extract of the supraoptic nucleus 1 hr after injection of [^{35}S]cysteine adjacent to this nucleus (solid line), and of labeled proteins in the above extract bound by anti-rat neurophysin antisera (broken line). Six percent polyacrylamide gels were used for isoelectric focusing; the sample buffer contained 8 M urea, 1% Triton X-100, and 2% ampholytes (pH 3–10); the sample was loaded at the anodal end of the gel. (From ref. 12).

Subsequent work[16-18] employing peptide mapping, affinity chromatography, and immunoprecipitation with vasopressin antisera after gentle tryptic digestion of the in vivo synthesized precursors provided evidence that these rat neurophysin precursors were indeed common precursors, as had been hypothesized by Sachs's group. In addition to identifying candidates for the vasopressin–neurophysin and oxytocin–neurophysin common precursors, these

---

FIGURE 2. Isoelectric focusing (pH 3–10 range ampholytes) of ^{35}S-labeled proteins extracted from the SONs of normal rats 20 min, 1 hr, 6 hr, and 24 hr after microinjecting [^{35}S]cysteine into the SON. The isoelectric points of the protein are indicated above each peak, and the position on the gels of a rat neurophysin standard is shown by the dotted line in the "24 hours" panel. (From ref. 13.)

studies also revealed that the vasopressin precursor (i.e., pro-pressophysin) was a glycoprotein (i.e., bound to concanavalin A columns), whereas the oxytocin precursor was not.[17] Consistent with this conclusion was the finding that a low-molecular-weight glycopeptide was transported to the posterior pituitary of normal but not homozygous Brattleboro rats.[17] From these data it was concluded that pro-pressophysin contained three peptide moieties: the vasopressin sequence, the vasopressin-associated neurophysin, and a <10,000-molecular-weight glycopeptide.

Such pulse–chase experiments in vivo, although classical in nature and generally less informative about the structures of the precursors than more modern approaches (see Sections 2.2 and 2.3), assist in the analysis of the molecular experiments. These studies can serve as a type of "quality control," showing that the amino acid sequences deduced by recombinant DNA techniques are indeed relevant to the actual precursor synthesized in situ. The order of peptide components in the in vivo synthesized pro-pressophysin (Pro-PP) and pro-oxyphysin (Pro-OP) molecules was suggested by the analysis of their cyanogen bromide cleavage products.[18] Pro-PP contains vasopressin at the N terminus, neurophysin in the middle, and the glycopeptide at the C terminus.[18] More careful analyses of the various pI forms of these precursors[18] indicated that both forms of Pro-PP (pI 5.6 and 6.1 in Figure 4) were of comparable molecular weight (about 19,000–20,000 daltons) and contained all of the known peptide products. We are uncertain whether the pI 5.6 form is an intermediate formed from the pI 6.1 form (Figure 4) or alternatively is a separate gene product differing in the glycopeptide moiety. In this regard, it is interesting that two distinct glycopeptides are transported to the pituitaries of normal rats, and that both are missing in Brattleboro rats.[17] Similarly we could not distinguish between the two forms of Pro-OP (pI 5.1 and 5.4 in Figure 4), both of which weigh about 15,000 daltons and appear to contain oxytocin and its neurophysin.[18] It will be interesting to see in future studies whether these multiple-pI forms of Pro-PP and Pro-OP observed in vivo are distinct gene products or consequences of posttranslational processing events.

2.2. Cell-Free Translation Studies

Several laboratories[19–22] have shown that mRNA isolated from bovine, mouse, or rat hypothalami could serve as templates in cell-free translation systems to yield 20,000–25,000-molecular-weight proteins, which could be

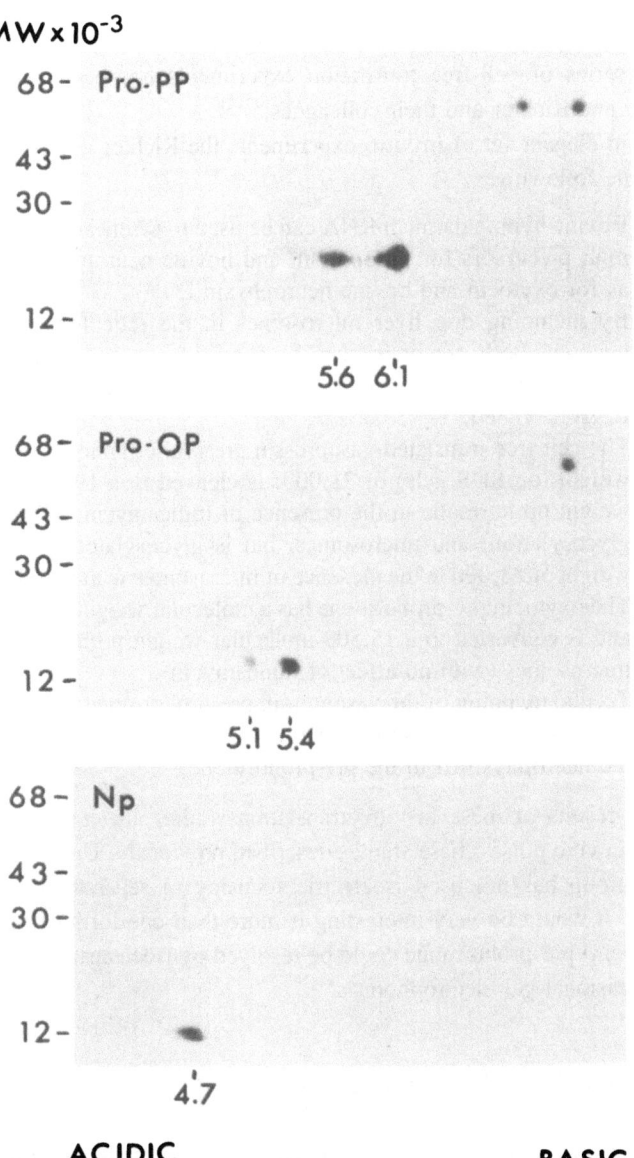

FIGURE 4. Two-dimensional gel electrophoresis and fluorography of [^{35}S]cysteine-labeled Pro-PP (top), Pro-OP (middle), and neurophysin (Np, bottom) synthesized by rat supraoptic nuclei and isolated by Sephadex G-75 chromatography. Insets show two-dimensional gels containing labeled Pro-PP and Pro-OP immunoprecipitated by antibodies to rat neurophysin. (From ref. 18.)

immunoprecipitated by antibodies raised against neurophysin. The most extensive series of cell-free translation experiments has been performed by Schmale and Richter and their colleagues.[22-28]

In an elegant set of in vitro experiments the Richter group has demonstrated the following:

1. Bovine hypothalamic mRNA can be used to synthesize separate common precursors for vasopressin and bovine neurophysin II, as well as for oxytocin and bovine neurophysin I.
2. By including dog liver microsomes in the reticulocyte translation cocktail, both precursors can be shown to be converted from pre-prohormones to prohormones, but only the vasopressin prohormone is glycosylated.
3. The cell-free translated vasopressin pre-prohormone has a molecular weight (on SDS gels) of 21,000, is cleaved to a 19,000-molecular-weight prohormone in the presence of tunicamycin (which prevents glycosylation) and microsomes, but is glycosylated to a molecular weight of 23,000 in the presence of microsomes without tunicamycin.
4. The oxytocin pre-prohormone has a molecular weight of about 16,500 and is converted to a 15,500-molecular-weight prohormone by liver microsomes (with no effect of tunicamycin).
5. Tryptic mapping of the vasopressin pre-prohormone and prohormone indicates that the vasopressin follows signal sequence and precedes the neurophysin II in the pre-prohormone.[22-28]

The results of these in vitro translation studies are entirely consistent with the in vivo pulse–chase studies described previously. Unfortunately, the Richter group has not used isoelectric focusing to separate the translated products. It would be very interesting if more than one form of vasopressin (or oxytocin) pre-prohormone could be resolved by isoelectric focusing or by two-dimensional gel electrophoresis.

2.3. Recombinant DNA Studies

Richter's group has recently reported the entire nucleotide sequence of cloned cDNA encoding the bovine vasopressin–neurophysin II pre-prohormone.[5] The corresponding aminoacid sequence contains 166 amino acids, of which 19 appear to belong to the signal sequence. The order of the peptide components in the prohormone is the same as that which was predicted from the in vivo and in vitro experiments described earlier. Figure 5 illustrates the

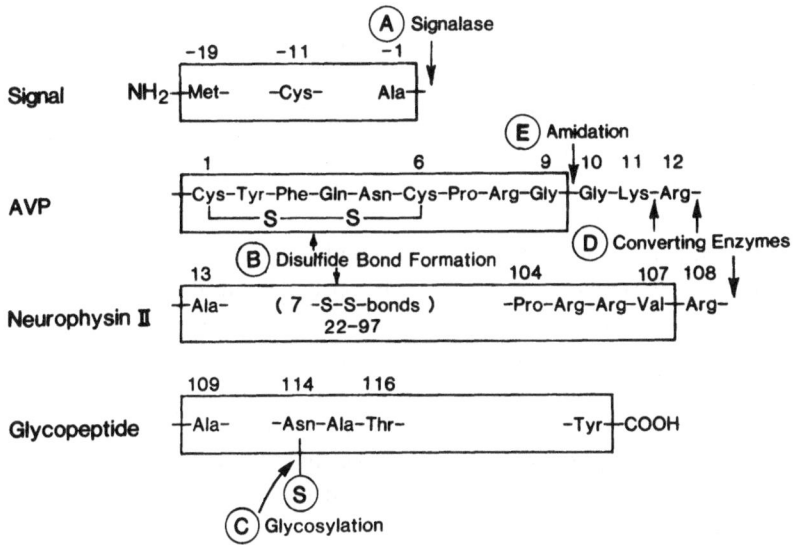

FIGURE 5. Structure of the bovine arginine–vasopressin–neurophysin II precursor. Arrows (A–E) denote posttranslational events occurring at specific sites on the precursor. (Modified from ref. 5.)

essential features of the vasopressin pre-prohormone elucidated by the recombinant DNA analysis.[5] The typical signal sequence (which begins with Met^{-19} at the N terminus, has a central hydrophobic region, and terminates with an amino acid with a small neutral side chain, i.e., Ala^{-1}) is immediately followed by the arginine vasopressin sequence, which is separated from the neurophysin II sequence by Gly^{10}-Lys^{11}-Arg^{12}, which in turn is separated from the 39-amino-acid C-terminal peptide by a single Arg^{108}. The latter 39-amino-acid peptide is believed to be the glycopeptide moiety discussed earlier, since it contains a characteristic amino acid sequence, Asn^{114}-Ala^{115}-Thr^{116}, typical of N-aspargine-linked glycopeptides.

There are both fulfilled expectations and some surprises in this sequence. As mentioned earlier, the order of peptide components was predicted from the previous in vivo and in vitro data. It was expected that the peptide components would be separated by basic amino acid residues since these are found in other prohormones, and owing to the results of previous tryptic mapping studies. However, while the Gly^{10}-Lys^{11}-Arg^{12} sequence interposed between vasopressin and neurophysin II is typical of prohormone cleavage sites where amidation also occurs, the single basic residue, Arg[108], between neurophysin II and the glycopeptide is not characteristic of other prohormone cleavage sites. These usually contain pairs of basic amino acids. Curiously, the Arg-Arg site in positions 105–106, which would appear to be more appropriate as a cleavage site, appears not to be recognized by the converting enzyme. These residues are found intact in bovine neurophysin II in situ.[15]

Perhaps the biggest surprise in this sequence was the identity of the 39-amino-acid putative glycopeptide. The complete amino acid sequence of the glycopeptide is shown in Table I. A glycopeptide with the identical amino acid sequence had previously been extracted from bovine pituitary, isolated, and sequenced by Smyth and Massey[29] in 1979. Similar glycopeptides with remarkable conservation of sequences were also found by these authors in pig and sheep pituitaries.[29] As these authors note in their paper, a similar 17-amino-acid glycopeptide (corresponding exactly to the 1–17 amino sequence in Table I, except that position 2 is Ser in the pig) had been isolated from pig posterior pituitary in 1972 by Holwerda.[30] Although the amino acid sequence of this glycopeptide had been known for some time, it was not until these recombinant DNA studies were done that it was associated with vasopressin biosynthesis. In addition to the 1–17 and 1–39 glycopeptide sequences, several other fragments were found (corresponding to sequences 1–10, 1–19, 23–39, and 26–39). While these have been interpreted as "naturally occurring" peptides,[29] it remains to be determined whether they are formed by the biosynthetic process (during posttranslational processing) in vivo, are natural degradative products, or are formed as a result of proteolytic

TABLE I. Amino Acid Sequence of the Glycopeptide in the Bovine Arginine Vasopressin–Neurophysin II Precursor[a]

1	3	10
NH₂-Ala-Asn-Asp-Arg-Ser-Asn-Ala-Thr-Leu-Leu-		
(109)	(113)	(118)
11	15	20
-Asp-Gly-Pro-Ser-Gly-Ala-Leu-Leu-Leu-Arg-		
(119)	(123)	(128)
21	25	30
-Leu-Val-Gln-Leu-Ala-Gly-Ala-Pro-Glu-Pro-		
(129)	(133)	(138)
31	35	39
-Ala-Glu-Pro-Ala-Gln-Pro-Gly-Val-Tyr-COOH		
(139)	(143)	(147)

[a] The amino acid order of the naturally found bovine glycopeptide[29] is shown numbered from 1 to 39; the numbers in parentheses show the corresponding positions in the prohormone.[5]

cleavages that occur during the isolation procedures. Only further pulse–chase-type studies performed in vivo will be able to resolve this issue.

2.4. Other Precursors for Vasopressin

In addition to the previously discussed possibility of multiple genes for the 20,000-molecular-weight arginine vasopressin precursor, there have been several claims of much larger arginine vasopressin and neurophysin precursors (i.e., around 80,000–140,000 daltons),[31–34] With regard to these reports, it is important to note that no in vivo and in vitro biosynthesis studies nor recombinant DNA studies supporting these claims have been reported. Until such experiments are published, one should remain open-minded but cautious about these larger putative precursors.

3. POSTTRANSLATIONAL PROCESSING OF THE ARGININE VASOPRESSIN–NEUROPHYSIN PRECURSOR

The previous sections outline the experimental evidence in support of the existance of the vasopressin precursor. However, knowing the complete sequence of a precursor is just one part of the story of the biosynthesis of the final peptide products. Of equal significance are the posttranslational processes that are involved in generating vasopressin, neurophysin, and the glycopeptide. The arrows in Figure 5 denote the expected processing events for the arginine vasopressin–neurophysin II precursor as deduced from its structure. The first three events, enzymatic cleavage of the signal peptide by a signalase, disulfide bond formation, and the initial stages of glycosylation, appear to occur during translation and are associated with the rough endoplasmic reticulum.[6–8] A second stage of glycosylation occurs within the Golgi apparatus.[6–8] The last two processes, enzymatic cleavage of the prohormone at the basic amino acid residues and amidation of the C-terminal glycine of vasopressin, appear to occur after packaging, within the secretory vesicles. Little is known about the nature of the enzymes involved in these processes.

Some insight as to the localization of the converting enzyme activity can be deduced from axonal transport studies.[11,14,35] These studies show that most of the precursor is transported into the axon, where it is converted to the final peptides during axonal transport.[11,14,35] Since the neurosecretory vesicles are the vesicles for the axonal transport of neurophysin and vasopressin, it would follow logically that these organelles are the sites of prohormone conversion. A similar proposal based on other data[4] had been put forth by the Sachs group, and localization of the conversion process in secretory vesicles has also been proposed in the biosynthesis of insulin, glucagon, and somatostatin in islet cells of the pancreas.[36,37]

Given the above hypothesis that the secretory vesicle is the major site for enzymatic cleavage of the prohormone, then one would expect that appropriate converting enzymes should be present in the vesicles. Recent experiments indicate that this is the case for a variety of tissues. Converting enzyme activity has been detected and partially characterized in secretory vesicles isolated from anglerfish pancreas islet cells,[36,37] neural and intermediate lobes of the rat pituitary,[38,39] and bovine posterior pituitary.[40] Analysis of the converting enzyme activities found in all of these secretory vesicles indicates that they are acid, thiol proteases with specificities of cleavage at pairs of basic amino acids.[36–40] Studies on the posttranslational processing enzymes are underway in a number of laboratories, and this promises to be a very active field of investigation in the near future.

4. FUTURE CONSIDERATIONS

The above discussion provides a summary of the progress in our understanding of the biosynthesis of vasopressin and neurophysin. With the complete sequencing of the bovine arginine vasopressin–neurophysin II precursor by recombinant DNA approaches, many new questions can now be addressed. One of these, the nature of posttranslational processing of the precursor, has already been discussed. Another pertains to the regulation of the biosynthesis of vasopressin. It is to be expected that radioactive cDNA probes for the precursor mRNA will soon be available. These will allow for the analysis of gene complexity and expression in vasopressin-synthesizing tissues (e.g., supraoptic nucleus, paraventricular nucleus, suprachiasmatic nucleus, tumors) under a variety of experimental conditions. Indeed it will be very interesting to employ these probes in an analysis of the genetic defect in the homozygous Brattleboro rat, as well as in investigating changes in gene expression in, for example, dehydration, lactation, and adrenalectomy. The discovery that vasopressin fibers emanating from paraventricular nucleus neurons project to many areas of the brain (see Chapter 2) raises the question of whether a family of vasopressin precursor genes exists, with differences in amino acid sequences in the C-terminal end (i.e., the glycopeptide region). It is conceivable that each of these neuronal pathways secretes a unique constellation of peptides, and that the peptides other than the vasopressin on these precursors are responsible for their biological activity. Indeed, the 39-amino-acid glycopeptide in the neural lobe itself requires further study as to its potential biological significance. A great deal has been learned over the past twenty years since Sachs and Takabatake[1,2] first suggested that a vasopressin precursor existed. However, it is also abundantly clear that we are still only at the threshold of understanding with respect to the biosynthesis of vasopressin and neurophysin, and further studies may alter our views about the biological significance of this precursor.

REFERENCES

1. Sachs, H, Takabatake Y: Evidence for a precursor in vasopressin biosynthesis. *Endocrinology* 75:943–948, 1964.
2. Takabatake Y, Sachs H: Vasopressin biosynthesis. III. *In vitro* studies. *Endocrinology* 75:934–942, 1964.
3. Fawcett CP, Powell AE, Sachs H: Biosynthesis and release of neurophysin. *Endocrinology* 83:1299–1310, 1968.
4. Sachs H, Fawcett P, Takabatake Y, et al: Biosynthesis and release of vasopressin and neurophysin. *Rec Prog Horm Res* 25: 447–491, 1969.
5. Land H, Schütz G, Schmale H, et al: Nucleotide sequence of cloned cDNA encoding bovine arginine vasopressin–neurophysin II precursor. *Nature* 295:299–303, 1982.
6. Zimmerman M, Mumford RA, Steiner DF (eds): Precursor processing in the biosynthesis of proteins. *Ann NY Acad Sci* 343:1–449, 1980.
7. Freedman RB, Hawkins HC (eds): *The Enzymology of Post-translational Modification of Proteins*. New York, Academic Press, 1980.
8. Koch G, Richter D (eds): *Biosynthesis, Modification, and Processing of Cellular and Viral Polyproteins*. New York, Academic Press, 1980.
9. Walter R, Audhya TK, Schlesinger DH, et al: Biosynthesis of neurophysin proteins in the dog and their isolation. *Endocrinology* 100:162–174, 1977.
10. Mendelson IS, Walter R: On the biosynthesis of putative neurophysin–vasopressin precursors in the hypothalamo-neurohypophysial gland of the guinea pig, in Voelter W, Gupta D (eds): *Hypothalamic Hormones*. Weinheim, Verlag Chemie, 1978.
11. Gainer H, Sarne Y, Brownstein MJ: Biosynthesis and axonal transport of rat neurohypophysial proteins and peptides. *J Cell Biol* 73:366–381, 1977.
12. Brownstein MJ, Robinson AG, Gainer H: Immunological identification of rat neurophysin precursors. *Nature* 269:259–261, 1977.
13. Brownstein MJ, Gainer H: Neurophysin biosynthesis in normal rats and in rats with hereditary diabetes insipidus. *Proc Natl Acad Sci USA* 74:4046–4049, 1977.

14. Gainer H, Brownstein MJ: Identification of the precursors of the rat neurophysins, in Vincent NJ, Kordon C (eds): *Cell Biology of Hypothalamic Neurosecretion*. Paris, CNRS, 1980.

15. Pickering BT, Jones CW: The neurophysins. *Horm Proteins Peptides* 5:103–158, 1978.

16. Russell JT, Brownstein MJ, Gainer H: Trypsin liberates an arginine vasopressin-like peptide and neurophysin from a M_r 20,000 putative common precursor. *Proc Natl Acad Sci USA* 76:6086-6090, 1979.

17. Russell JT, Brownstein MJ, Gainer H: Biosynthesis of vasopressin, oxytocin, and neurophysins: Isolation and characterization of two common precursors (propressophysin and prooxyphysin). *Endocrinology* 107:1880–1891, 1980.

18. Russell JT, Brownstein MJ, Gainer H: Biosynthesis of neurohypophyseal polypeptides: The order of peptide components in propressophysin and prooxyphysin. *Neuropeptides* 2:59–65, 1981.

19. Guidice LC, Chaiken IM: Immunological and chemical identification of a neurophysin-containing protein coded by messenger RNA from bovine hypothalamus. *Proc Natl Acad Sci USA* 70:3800–3804, 1979.

20. Guidice LM, Chaiken IM: Cell-free biosynthesis of different high molecular forms of bovine neurophysin I and II coded by hypothalamic mRNA. *J Biol Chem* 254:11767–11770, 1979.

21. Lin C, Joseph-Bravo P, Sherman T, et al: Cell-free synthesis of putative neurophysin precursors from rat and mouse hypothalamic poly(A)-RNA. *Biochem Biophys Res Commun* 89:943–950, 1979.

22. Schmale H, Leipold B, Richter D: Cell-free translation of bovine hypothalamic mRNA: Synthesis and processing of the preproneurophysins I and II. *FEBS Lett* 108:311–316, 1979.

23. Richter D, Schmale H, Ivell R, et al: Hypothalamic mRNA-directed synthesis of neuropeptides: Immunological identification of precursors to neurophysin II/arginine vasopressin and to neurophysin I/oxytocin, in Kock G, Richter D (eds): *Biosynthesis, Modification, and Processing of Cellular and Viral Polyproteins*. New York, Academic Press, 1980.

24. Schmale H, Richter D: *In vitro* biosynthesis and processing of composite common precursors containing amino acid sequences identified immunologically as neurophysin I/oxytocin and as neurophysin II/vasopressin. *FEBS Lett* 121:358–362, 1980.

25. Ivell R, Schmale H, Richter D: Glycosylation of the arginine vasopressin/neurophysin II common precursor. *Biochem Biophys Res Commun* 102:1230–1236, 1981.

26. Schamle H, Richter D: Immunological identification of a common precursor to arginine vasopressin and neurophysin II synthesized by *in vitro* translation of bovine hypothalamic mRNA. *Proc Natl Acad Sci USA* 78:766–769, 1981.

27. Schmale H, Richter D: A direct comparison of the rat and bovine arginine vasopressin/neurophysin II common precursor. *Neuropeptides* 2:151–156, 1981.

28. Schmale H, Richter D: Tryptic release of authentic arginine vasopressin$_{1-8}$ from a composite arginine vasopressin/neurophysin II precursor. *Neuropeptides* 2:47–52, 1981.

29. Smyth DG, Massey DE: A new glycopeptide in pig, ox, and sheep pituitary. *Biochem Biophys Res Commun* 87:1006–1010, 1979.

30. Holwerda DA: A glycopeptide from the posterior lobe of pig pituitaries. 2. Primary structure. *Eur J Biochem* 28:340–346, 1972.

31. Lauber M, Camier M, Cohen P: Immunological and biochemical characterization of distinct high molecular weight forms of neurophysin and somatostatin in mouse hypothalamus extracts. *FEBS Lett* 97:343–347, 1979.

32. Camier M, Lauber M, Mohring J, et al: Evidence for higher molecular weight immunoreactive forms of vasopressin in the mouse hypothalamus. *FEBS Lett* 108:369–373, 1979.

33. Lauber M, Nicolas P, Boussetta H, et al: The M_r 80,000 common forms of neurophysin and vasopressin from bovine neurohypophysis have corticotropin- and β-endorphin-like

sequences and liberate by proteolysis biologically active corticotropin. *Proc Natl Acad Sci USA* 78:6086–6090, 1981.

34. Beguin P, Nicolas P, Bousetta H, et al: Characterization of the 80,000 molecular weight form of neurophysin isolated from bovine neurohypophysis. *J Biol Chem* 256:9289–9294, 1981.

35. Gainer H, Sarne Y, Brownstein JJ: Neurophysin biosynthesis: Conversion of a putative precursor during axonal transport. *Science* 195:1354–1356, 1977.

36. Fletcher DJ, Noe BD, Bauer GE, et al: Characterization of the conversion of a somatostatin precursor to somatostatin by islet secretory granules. *Diabetes* 29:593–599, 1980.

37. Fletcher DJ, Quigley JP, Bauer GE, et al: Characterization of pro-insulin and pro-glucagon converting activities in isolated secretory granules. *J Cell Biol* 90:312–322, 1981.

38. Loh YP, Gainer H: Characterization of pro-opiocortin converting activity in purified secretory granules from rat pituitary neurointermediate lobe. *Proc Natl Acad Sci USA* 79:108–112, 1982.

39. Loh YP, Chang TL: Pro-opiocortin converting activity in rat intermediate and neural lobe secretory granules, *FEBS Lett* 127:57–62, 1982.

40. Change TL, Gainer H, Russell JT, et al: Proopiocortin converting enzyme activity in bovine neurosecretory granules. *Endocrinology* 111:1607–1614, 1982.

4

THE MODE OF ACTION OF ANTIDIURETIC HORMONE
Membrane Reorganization, Recycling, and Intracellular Transport

David B. P. Goodman and Walter Davis

1. HISTORICAL BACKGROUND

The discovery of the antidiuretic effect of posterior pituitary extracts was made by two physicians, Francesco Farini, a Venetian,[1] and R. von den Velden, a German.[2] Both clinicians had been impressed with the strong evidence of a connection between the occurrence of diabetes insipidus and diseases (tumors, syphilis, tuberculosis) and lesions of the pituitary gland. These observations suggested the possibility that pituitary hypofunction might be alleviated by the administration of posterior pituitary extracts to patients with diabetes insipidus. Farini[1] reported on two patients with daily urine volumes of 5–6 and 7.5–8 liters respectively. In both cases injection of posterior pituitary extract decreased urine volume dramatically, down to 2–3 liters/day. Von den Velden[2] described the treatment of a patient with idiopathic diabetes insipidus. Administration of subcutaneous injections of posterior pituitary extracts caused the patient's urine specific gravity to rise from 1.005 to 1.010 and his 24-hr urine volume to fall from 6 to less than 3 liters. Additionally, von den Velden showed that water diuresis in healthy individuals was inhibited by pituitary extract. These observations were quickly confirmed

David B. P. Goodman • Department of Pathology and Laboratory Medicine, University of Pennsylvania Medical School, Philadelphia, Pennsylvania 19104. **Walter Davis** • Department of Microscopic Anatomy, Baylor College of Dentistry, Dallas, Texas 75246.

by others (for references see ref. 3). However, the most important study on the mechanism of the antidiuretic effect of posterior pituitary extracts was that of Starling and Verney,[4] who in 1924 demonstrated an antidiuretic effect of posterior pituitary extracts on the isolated kidney. It was also shown that when kidneys were damaged by cantharides or a uranium salt, the usually observed polyuria was not inhibited by pituitary extracts.[5]

It soon became clear that when small amounts of antidiuretic hormone (ADH) are injected into a mammal in water diuresis, urine volume decreases and osmolality increases. Urine osmolality may even exceed plasma osmolality. If the mammal is dehydrated the urine flow will fall even lower and will certainly become hyperosmotic relative to plasma. Under these circumstances the glomerular filtration rate and total solute excretion do not change. That ADH acts on the distal portion of the mammalian kidney was first suggested by Smith[6] and associates[7] to account for the reduction in solute-free water excretion that followed hormone administration during osmotic diuresis. Further studies presented additional evidence to support this site for the hormone-elicited change in water permeability,[8–10] as well as a similar effect of the hormone on the permeability of the distal nephron to urea.[11–13] Subsequently direct studies of the isolated perfused collecting tubule of the rabbit[14] and the medullary collecting ducts of the rat[15] established the effect of the hormone at these distal sites.

To understand how ADH or dehydration brings about water conservation requires that a distinction be made between the two major components of the total mammalian antidiuretic response.[16] The first component is a change in tubular water permeability, which allows tubular fluids to come into osmotic equilibrium with the peritubular fluids. The second component allows the urine to become hyperosmotic with reference to the plasma. This is possible if the osmolality of the interstitial fluids in some part of the kidney is higher than that in plasma. Osmotic equilibrium between tubular urine and the hypertonic interstitium would also be facilitated if ADH increased water permeability in those segments exposed to hyperosmotic peritubular fluids.

2. THE TOAD URINARY BLADDER AS A MODEL SYSTEM

Because of the anatomical complexity and cellular heterogeneity of the mammalian kidney, detailed analysis of the mechanism of action of ADH has been carried out in a simpler model system, the toad urinary bladder. This tissue responds to ADH much as does the distal mammalian nephron.[17-19] There are differences concerning permeability to solutes and effects on ion transport, but the changes in osmotic permeability to water are similar.[14]

The toad urinary bladder is a thin-walled bilobed structure consisting of a single layer of transport epithelial cells supported by a loose connective tissue. The tissue survives in vitro for up to 48 hr and is extremely resistant to mechanical and chemical manipulations. In the absence of ADH the luminal or urinary membrane of the epithelial cell layer is highly impermeable to water. Upon addition of ADH the water permeability of this membrane increases 30- to 50-fold and bulk water movement down an imposed osmotic gradient can be easily measured gravimetrically.[17]

3. THE BIOCHEMICAL MODE OF ANTIDIURETIC HORMONE ACTION

Detailed evidence for the molecular mode of ADH action began to be presented in the early 1960s. It was initially demonstrated that exogenous cyclic AMP (cAMP) and phosphodiesterase inhibitors could mimic the hydroosmotic effect of ADH as well as the effects of the hormone on solute permeability in the toad bladder.[20,21] Subsequently, it was shown that ADH addition caused an increase in the cAMP content of the toad bladder[22] and that phosphodiesterase inhibitors could mimic the effect of ADH. Additionally, a hormone-sensitive adenylate cyclase in a plasma-membrane-enriched subcellular fraction[23] and cAMP-dependent protein kinases[24] were both described and characterized. These experimental data established cAMP as a second messenger in the action of ADH (Table I).

ADH can be thought to act initially by interacting with specific receptors in the basolateral or serosal plasma membrane of the epithelial cells. This

TABLE I. Experimental Evidence for the Molecular Mode of ADH Action

1. ADH increases tissue cAMP content.
2. Theophylline and other phosphodiesterase inhibitors enhance the response to ADH.
3. Exogenous cAMP mimics the response to ADH.
4. An ADH-sensitive adenylate cyclase is localized in a membrane fraction of the tissue.
5. cAMP-dependent protein kinases are present in the tissue.

hormone–receptor interaction causes adenylate cyclase activation and the accumulation of cAMP. The rise in cAMP leads to protein kinase activation and the phosphorylation of one or more protein substrates at the luminal membrane of the epithelial cells. This phosphorylation is postulated to be involved in the change in luminal membrane water permeability (Figure 1). Direct experimental evidence to support this postulate has not been provided. Support for this model of ADH action has, however, been presented by Schwartz and co-workers.[25] These workers succeeded in separating and isolating luminal and basolateral plasma membranes from epithelial cells of the bovine renal papillae, an ADH-sensitive position of that organ. In these isolated membrane fractions the ADH-stimulated adenylate cyclase was predominantly associated with the basolateral membrane and the luminal membrane contained a cAMP-dependent protein kinase that catalyzed the phosphorylation of protein substrates in the luminal membrane.

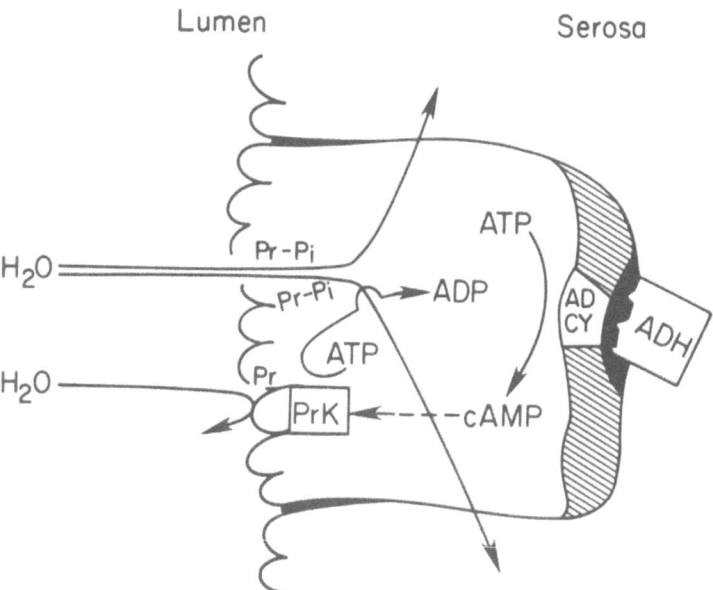

FIGURE 1. A model for the action of ADH on water permeability. The peptide hormone binds to its receptor in the serosal membrane. This hormone–receptor interaction leads to stimulation of adenylate cyclase and the consequent increase in the concentration of cAMP in the tissue. cAMP then activates a protein kinase in the luminal membrane. The activated protein kinase catalyzes the phosphorylation of specific membrane protein(s) that function in altering the water permeability of the membrane.

4. THE PERMEABILITY OF THE LUMINAL MEMBRANE

As mentioned in Section 3, no direct evidence has been presented indicating that the phosphorylation of specific membrane proteins leads to a change in luminal membrane water permeability. Considerable evidence has, however, been presented that indicates that a reorganization in the structure of the luminal membrane accompanies the change in membrane water permeability.[26]

When examined by freeze–fracture electron microscopy the luminal membrane of the toad urinary bladder has been shown to possess intramembrane particles, which represent membrane proteins intercalated within the membrane lipid bilayer. These particles are not unique to the toad bladder since nearly all biological membranes have this appearance when examined by freeze–fracture microscopy. In the absence of ADH the intramembrane particles are randomly distributed in an apparently homogeneous matrix. After ADH treatment the intramembrane particles are found in organized aggregates. Within these aggregates the individual particles appear in linear arrays (Figure 2). While the exact meaning of the structural change observed after ADH treatment is not known, the observation of organization is potentially important since it suggests that these structures are not random aggregates but may represent a specific reorganization of membrane structure.[27–30]

The question arises as to whether these membrane aggregates represent the actual site of the permeability change or whether they represent a secondary effect caused by the permeability change. This question is quickly resolved by the observation that the structural change in the luminal membrane still occurs in bladder exposed to hormone in the absence of an osmotic gradient, i.e., where there is no osmotic water flow.[29,30] Additional evidence has been reported showing a quantitative correlation between the frequency of membrane aggregates and the rate of osmotic water flow.[31] Other data indicate that the aggregates are specifically associated with the increase in water permeability. Aggregates are present in the luminal membrane during hydroosmotic response to serosal hypertonicity,[29] a condition that depresses transepithelial sodium transport, and methohexital, an anesthetic that inhibits water permeability selectively without reducing urea and sodium permeability, reduces the number of aggregates induced by ADH.[32] These particles are not unique to the amphibian urinary bladder, since comparable structures have been observed in such other ADH-sensitive tissues as mammalian collecting ducts[33] and toad skin.[34]

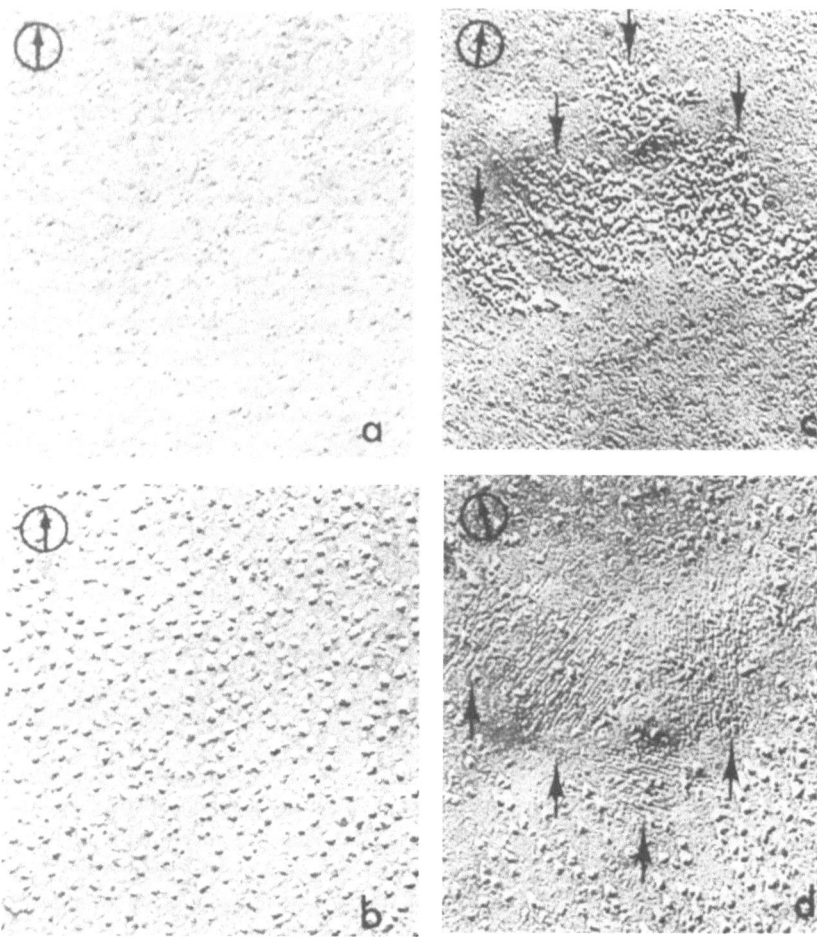

FIGURE 2. Freeze–fracture electron micrographs of toad bladder epithelial cell luminal membrane in the absence (a,b) or presence (c,d) of ADH. Inner (a) and outer (b) fracture faces from tissue without ADH stimulation demonstrate intramembranous particles that are not aggregated. The inner fracture face after ADH treatment (c) shows separate sites of aggregated intramembranous particles (single arrows). The outer fracture face after ADH treatment (d), which is complementary to (c), shows organized linear arrays of depressions corresponding to the aggregated intramembranous particles shown in (c) (single arrows). Circled arrows indicate shadowing direction. 83,000 ×. (From ref. 28.)

If these aggregates are the actual site of water flow, then the source of this intramembranous complex becomes of great interest. Several possible hypotheses have been presented to explain the source of the aggregates: The aggregates may form from material already present in the membrane by reorganization, reassociation, or realignment of individual intramembrane particles. Alternatively the aggregates may result from insertion of new material into the luminal membrane or from insertion of individual particles that are subsequently assembled within the membrane into aggregates. Finally, the aggregates might exist preassembled in cytoplasmic membranes and fuse with the luminal membrane as part of the ADH-induced change in water permeability. Evidence accumulated to date supports this last hypothesis.

When the toad bladder is examined early in the response to ADH, before water flow is maximal, careful analysis demonstrates that mean aggregate size is not smaller and that the frequency of small aggregates is not increased compared to control tissue.[35] However, aggregates with organization identical to that found in the luminal membrane of hormone-treated tissue are found in cytoplasmic vacuoles[36] and the number of these vacuoles with aggregates falls by approximately 50% after ADH treatment.[37,38] These data have led to the formulation of the *membrane shuttle hypothesis* to explain the action of ADH on apical or luminal membrane water permeability.[31,38] In the absence of ADH the luminal membrane is impermeable to water. With the addition of hormone the aggregate-containing membrane is translocated to and fuses with the luminal membrane. This fusion results in a marked increase in the water permeability of the membrane. This membrane shuttle hypothesis implies that the organized aggregates serve as a mechanism to provide channels for water flow within restricted areas of the membrane (Figure 3).

5. BASIS FOR SUSTAINED WATER MOVEMENT

The membrane shuttle hypothesis provides an explanation for the change in luminal membrane water permeability induced by ADH. However, there are two experimental maneuvers, alteration in ionic composition of the serosal bathing solution[39] and treatment of the toad bladder with the macrolide antibiotic cytochalasin B,[40] which dissociate the change in luminal water permeability induced by ADH from sustained bulk water movement. The data, which will be reviewed subsequently, indicate that additional cellular mech-

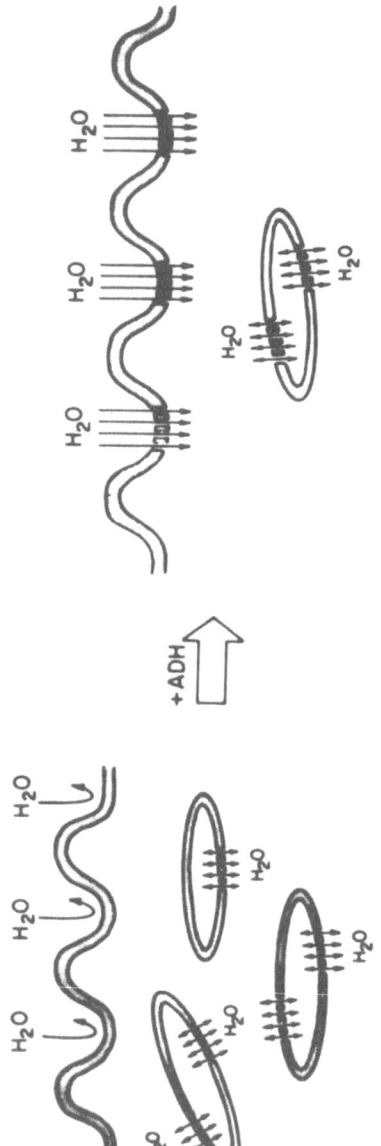

FIGURE 3. The membrane shuttle hypothesis. Portions of membrane highly permeable to water are shuttled from cytoplasmic vacuoles to the luminal plasma membrane upon addition of ADH, leading to enhanced membrane water permeability. These areas of membrane with high water permeability are thought to be represented as intramembrane particle aggregates when the membrane is examined by freeze–fracture electron microscopy. (From ref. 38.)

anisms operating distal to the change in luminal water permeability are required to support the complete sustained hydroosmotic response to ADH.

When either serosal sodium or serosal potassium is replaced isosmotically with either choline or sucrose, the hydroosmotic response to ADH is reduced by approximately 50%.[39] This reduction in response is not accompanied by any alteration in the increase in the hormone-induced diffusion of ^3H_2O across the tissue, a response that is the usual measure of luminal membrane water permeability. Since the inhibitory effect of monovalent cation replacement is observed even when an exogenous cAMP derivative is used to induce the hydroosmotic response, it is unlikely that the effect of serosal monovalent alteration on the hydroosmotic response to ADH is due simply to an alteration in cAMP generation or compartmentation. The ionic replacements employed do not cause inhibition of the hydroosmotic response through an inhibition of the Na^+,K^+-ATPase since ouabain, a potent inhibitor of transepithelial Na^+ transport in the toad bladder,[41] has no effect on the hydroosmotic response to ADH.

Cytochalasin B, a fungal antibiotic that interferes with the function of cellular microfilaments,[42] produces a pattern of inhibition of the hydroosmotic response in the toad bladder similar to the effect of monovalent cation replacement described previously, i.e., the magnitude of the increase in bulk water flow induced by ADH is inhibited by about 50%, but the change in luminal membrane water permeability as measured by ^3H_2O diffusion is not affected.[40] Under these conditions cytochalasin causes the formation of large intracellular vacuoles or lakes, which contain electron-dense precipitates when the tissue is fixed with pyroantimonate.[43] This fixation procedure is used routinely to demonstrate cation accumulation at the electron microscopic level.

An explanation for the effect of cation replacement and cytochalasin on the response to ADH can be proposed when one considers recent morphologic evidence demonstrating an effect of ADH on vesicular activity at the basal and lateral aspects of the epithelial cells in the toad bladder.[44] In the control tissue fixed in the presence of an osmotic gradient, vesicles are evident along the basal aspect of the epithelial cell layer and along the plicated lateral cell borders between adjacent epithelial cells. After ADH addition the number of vesicles increases about threefold (Figure 4). In control epithelial cells the mean area occupied by vesicles was $0.92 \pm 0.15\%$ of the total cytoplasmic areas as compared to $2.67 \pm 0.39\%$ after hormone-induced hydroosmotic water flow. When the toad bladder is examined at frequent time intervals after ADH addition, it can be seen that cytochalasin does not prevent the

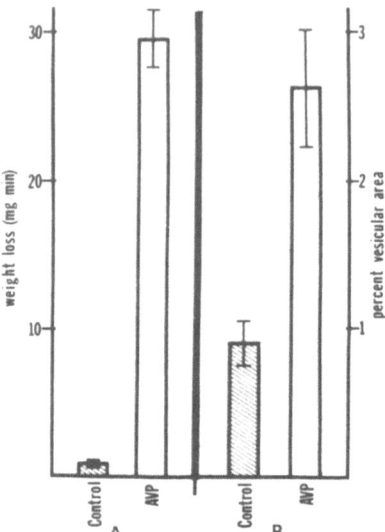

FIGURE 4. The effect of ADH on hydroosmotic water flow (A) and the percentage of cellular area at the serosal and lateral aspect of toad bladder epithelial cells occupied by vesicles (B) in the presence and absence of antidiuretic hormone (AVP).

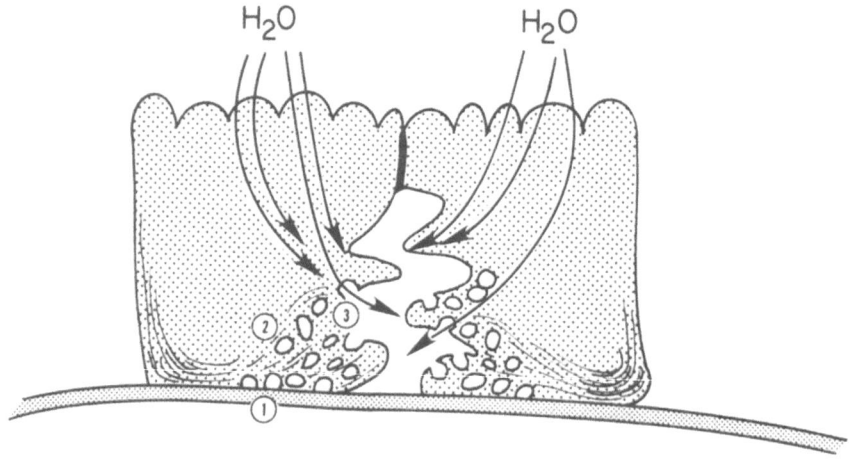

FIGURE 5. The translocation of osmotically active material from the basal aspect of epithelial cells to the lateral intercellular space. Vesicles form at the basal aspect of cells (1) and are transported to the lateral intercellular plications (2), and the osmotically active material is released after exocytosis (3) into the lateral intercellular space to provide osmotically active material to sustain hydroosmotic water flow.

increase in vesicular activity induced by the hormone.[43] Cytochalasin does, however, cause an increase in the formation of multivesicular bodies, possibly interfering with the lateral migration of single vesicles, a process that may require an interplay between membranes and microfilaments. Since the basally derived vesicles and the multivesicular bodies contain sodium and/or other osmotically active materials, these intracellular organelles are hypertonic, and, since the apical membrane water permeability is increased by ADH, the multivesicular bodies accumulate water and swell. Eventually large intracellular lakes are formed. The net effect is a diminished hydroosmotic response.

The traversing of vesicles from one side of a cell to the other is known to occur in a variety of cell types.[45–47] In the case of the toad urinary bladder epithelium one can hypothesize that these vesicles function to shuttle osmotically active materials (sodium) from the basal or serosal aspect of the epithelium to the lateral intercellular space. Once released by exocytosis at this location, the osmotically active materials would serve to create and renew the necessary osmotic gradients required for the sustained hydroosmotic water flow, i.e., salt–water coupling (Figure 5).

6. PROSPECTIVE

In this review we have attempted to point out new aspects of ADH action that have been proposed to involve membrane reorganization, recycling, and intracellular transport. In the case of both the change in luminal membrane water permeability and the distal intracellular mechanism necessary for sustained hydroosmotic water flow, evidence to support such mechanisms has been reported. This evidence, which is largely morphologic and circumstantial, must now be corroborated by independent biochemical approaches. In these biochemical studies the role of cAMP and protein phosphorylation must clearly be evaluated. One might think that a unique mechanism has evolved for the action of ADH, but recent evidence points to analogous responses in the action of insulin. Insulin's stimulation of carbohydrate transport into cells results from an alteration in the content of carbohydrate carriers in the plasma membrane induced by the transfer of these carriers from intracellular membranes to the plasma membrane.[48,49] These findings suggest that additional common mechanisms for peptide hormone action, in addition to the widely acknowledged cAMP–protein kinase system, may exist.

REFERENCES

1. Farini F: Diabete insipido ed opoterapia. *Gazz Osped Clin* 34:1135–1139, 1913.
2. Von den Velden R: Die Nierenwirkung von Hypophysenextrakten beim menschen. *Klin Wochenschr* 50:2083–2086, 1913.
3. Thorn NA: The influence of the neurohypophyseal hormones and similar peptides on the kidneys, in Berde B (ed): *Handbook of Experimental Pharmacology: Neurohypophyseal Hormones and Similar Polypeptides*. Berlin, Springer-Verlag, 1968, vol 23, pp. 372–442.
4. Starling EH, Verney EB: The secretion of urine as studied on the isolated kidney. *Proc R Soc London Ser B* 97:321–363, 1924.
5. Molitor H, Pick EP: Zur Kenntnis der Pituitrin Wirkung auf die Diurese. *Arch Exp Pathol Pharmakol* 101:180–194, 1924.
6. Smith HW: *The Kidney: Structure and Function in Health and Disease*. Fairlawn, New Jersey, Oxford, 1951, p 329.
7. Wesson LG Jr, Anslow WP Jr: Effect of osmotic and mercurial diuresis on simultaneous water diuresis. *Am J Physiol* 170:255–269, 1952.
8. Gottschalk CW, Mylie M: Micropuncture study of the mammalian urinary concentrating mechanism: Evidence for the counter current hypothesis. *Am J Physiol* 196:927–936, 1969.
9. Ullrich KJ, Rumrich G, Fuchs G: Wasserpermeabilität und transtubulärer Wasserfluss corticales Nephronabschnitte bei verschiedenen Diuresezuständin. *Arch Ges Physiol* 280:99–119, 1964.
10. Wirz H: Der osmotische Druck in den corticalen Tubuli der Rattenniere. *Helv Physiol Pharmacol Acta* 14:353–363, 1956.
11. Aukland K: Renal tubular permeability to urea with special reference to accumulation of urea in the renal medulla. *Scand J Clin Lab Invest* 13:646–660, 1961.
12. Capek KG, Fuchs G, Rumrich G, et al: Harnstoffpermeabilität der corticalen Tubulusabschnitte von Ratten in Antidiurese und Wasserdiurese. *Arch Ges Physiol* 290:237–249, 1966.
13. Jaenike JR: Influence of Vasopressin on the permeability of the mammalian collecting duct to urea. *J Clin Invest* 30:144–151, 1961.
14. Grantham JJ, Burg MB: Effect of vasopressin and cyclic AMP on permeability of isolated collecting tubules. *Am J Physiol* 211:255–259, 1966.
15. Morgan TF, Sakai F, Berliner RW: In vitro permeability of medullary collecting ducts to water and urea. *Am J Physiol* 214:574–581, 1968.
16. Sawyer WH: The mammalian antidiuretic response, in Knobil E, Sawyer WH (eds): *Handbook of Physiology*, Section 7: *Endocrinology*. Washington DC, American Physiological Society, 1974, vol IV, pt 1, chap 16, pp 443–468.
17. Bentley PJ: The effects of neurohypophyseal extracts on water transfer across the wall of isolated urinary bladder of the toad *Bufo marinus*. *J Endocrinol* 17:201–209, 1958.
18. Maffly RH, Hays RM, Lamdin E, et al: The effect of neurohypophyseal hormones on the permeability of the toad bladder to urea. *J Clin Invest* 39:630–641, 1960.
19. Sawyer WH: Increased water permeability of the bullfrog (*Rana catesbeiana*) bladder in vitro in response to synthetic oxytocin and arginine vasotocin and to neurohypophyseal extracts from nonmammalian vertebrates. *Endocrinology* 66:112–120, 1960.
20. Orloff J, Handler JS: Vasopressin-like effects of adenosine 3′, 5′-phosphate (cyclic 3′,5′-AMP) and theophylline in the toad bladder. *Biochem Biophys Res Commun* 5:63–66, 1961.
21. Orloff J, Handler JS: The similarity of effects of vasopressin, adenosine 3′,5′-phosphate (cyclic AMP) and theophylline on the toad bladder. *J Clin Invest* 41:702–709, 1962.

22. Handler JS, Butcher RW, Sutherland EW, et al: The effect of vasopressin and of theophylline on the concentration of adenosine $3',5'$-phosphate in the urinary bladder of the toad. *J Biol Chem* 240:4524–4526, 1965.

23. Bar HP, Hechter O, Schwartz IL, et al: Neurohypophyseal hormone-sensitive adenyl-cyclase of toad urinary bladder. *Proc Natl Acad Sci USA* 67:7–12, 1970.

24. Kirchberger MA, Schwartz IL, Walter R: Cyclic $3',5'$-AMP-dependent protein kinase activity in toad bladder epithelium. *Proc Soc Exp Biol Med* 140:657–660, 1972.

25. Schwartz IL, Schlatz LJ, Kinne-Saffran E, et al: Target cell polarity and membrane phosphorylation in relation to the mechanism of action of antidiuretic hormone. *Proc Natl Acad Sci USA* 71:2595–2599, 1974.

26. Wade JB, Kachadorian WA, DiScala VA: Freeze–fracture electron microscopy: Relationship of membrane structural features to transport physiology. *Am J Physiol* 232:F77–F83, 1977.

27. Chevalier J, Bourguet J, Hugon JS: Membrane associated particles: Distribution in frog urinary bladder epithelium at rest and after oxytocin treatment. *Cell Tissue Res* 152:129–140, 1974.

28. Kachadorian WA, Wade JB, DiScala VA: Vasopressin: Induced structural change in toad bladder luminal membrane. *Science* 190:67–69, 1975.

29. Bourguet J, Chevalier J, Hugon JS: Alterations in membrane-associated particle distribution during antidiuretic challenge in frog urinary bladder epithelium. *Biophys J* 16:627–639, 1976.

30. Kachadorian WA, Wade JB, Uiterwyk CC, et al: Membrane structural and functional responses to vasopressin in toad bladder. *J Membr Biol* 30:381–401, 1977.

31. Wade JB, Stetson DL, Lewis SA: ADH action: Evidence for a membrane shuttle mechanism. *Ann NY Acad Sci* 372:106–117, 1981.

32. Kachadorian WA, Levine SD, Wade JB, et al: Relationship of aggregated intramembranous particles to water permeability in vasopressin-treated toad urinary bladder. *J Clin Invest* 59:576–581, 1977.

33. Harmanci MC, Kachadorian WA, Valtin H, et al: Antidiuretic hormone-induced intramembranous alterations in mammalian collecting ducts. *Am J Physiol* 235:F440–F443, 1978.

34. Brown D, Grosso A, DeSousa RC: Isoproterenol-induced intramembranous particle aggregation and water flux in toad epidermis. *Biochim Biophys Acta* 596:158–164, 1980.

35. Kachadorian WA, Casey C, DiScala VA: Time course of ADH-induced intramembranous particle aggregation in toad urinary bladder. *Am J Physiol* 234:F461–F465, 1978.

36. Muller J, Kachadorian WA, DiScala VA: Evidence that ADH-stimulated intramembrane particle aggregates are transferred from cytoplasmic to luminal membranes in toad bladder epithelial cells. *J Cell Biol* 85:83–95, 1980.

37. Wade JB: Hormonal modulation of epithelial structure. *Curr Top Membr Transp* 13:123–147, 1980.

38. Wade JB: Modulation of membrane structure in the toad urinary bladder by vasopressin, in Ussing HH, Bindslev N, Lassen NA, et al (eds): *Water Transport Across Epithelia*, Alfred Benzon Symposia, vol 15. Copenhagen, Munksgaard, 1981, pp 422–436.

39. Davis WL, Goodman DBP, Rasmussen H: Ionic and metabolic requirements for the hydroosmotic response to antidiuretic hormone in toad urinary bladder. *J Membr Biol* 41:225–239, 1978.

40. Davis WL, Goodman DBP, Schuster RJ, et al: Effects of cytochalasin B on the response of toad urinary bladder to vasopressin. *J Cell Biol* 63:986–997, 1974.

41. Goodman DBP, Allen JE, Rasmussen H: On the mechanism of action of aldosterone. *Proc Natl Acad Sci USA* 64:330–337, 1969.

42. Wessels NK, Spooner BS, Ash JF, et al: Microfilaments in cellular and developmental processes. *Science* 171:135–143, 1971.

43. Davis WL, Jones RG, Hagler HK, et al: Intracellular water transport in the action of ADH. *Ann NY Acad Sci* 372:118–130, 1981.

44. Davis WL, Jones RG, Ciumei J, et al: An electron microscopic and morphometric study of vesiculation in the toad urinary bladder epithelial cell layer: Effect of antidiuretic hormone. *Cell Tissue Res* 225:619–631, 1982.

45. Bruns RR, Palade GE: Studies on blood capillaries. II. Transport of ferritin molecules across the wall of muscle capillaries. *J Cell Biol* 37:277–299, 1968.

46. Rodewall R: Intestinal transport of antibodies in the newborn rat. *J Cell Biol* 58:189–211, 1973.

47. Hill AE: General mechanisms of salt–water coupling in epithelia, in Gupta BL, Moreton RB, Oschman JL, et al (eds): *Transport of Ions and Water in Animals*. New York, Academic Press, 1977, pp 183–214.

48. Suzuki K, Kono T: Evidence that insulin causes translocation of glucose transport activity to the plasma membrane from an intracellular storage site. *Proc Natl Acad Sci USA* 77:2542–2545, 1980.

49. Karnieli E, Zarnowski MJ, Hissin PJ, et al: Insulin-stimulated translocation of glucose transport systems in the isolated rat adipose cell: Time course, reversal, insulin concentration dependency, and relationship to glucose transport activity. *J Biol Chem* 256:4772–4777, 1981.

5

THE CONTRIBUTION OF MEASURED SECRETION OF NEUROPHYSINS TO OUR UNDERSTANDING OF NEUROHYPOPHYSIAL FUNCTION

Alan G. Robinson

1. BACKGROUND

When biologically active peptides were first extracted from posterior pituitaries, the active principle was thought to be a 30,000-molecular-weight protein, the Van Dyke protein, which possessed both oxytocin and vasopressin bioactivity.[1,2] In 1956 Acher and his colleagues,[3-5] working in Paris, demonstrated that when the Van Dyke protein was subjected to changes in pH and electrodialysis in solution two biologically active hormones, vasopressin and oxytocin, were reversibly separated from a carrier protein. The carrier protein was named *neurophysine*. Specific bioassay techniques were then developed for the two hormones, and the basic physiologic function of the posterior pituitary peptides was described over the next several years.[6,7]

In recent years interest has focused again upon the neurophysins for three reasons: (1) Separate and specific neurophysins for vasopressin and for oxytocin can be identified in several species; (2) a specific neurophysin is secreted with its respective hormone at all sites of hormone release; and (3) a specific neurophysin is part of a precursor molecule for its respective hormone. Each

---

Alan G. Robinson ● University of Pittsburgh School of Medicine, Pittsburgh, Pennsylvania 15261.

of these three areas of investigation was initiated by biochemical studies of neurophysins and each has also been greatly aided by the development of specific antibodies reactive with individual neurophysins. It is fortunate for studies of neurohypophysial function that the neurophysins are much more antigenic than the hormones of the posterior pituitary, and numerous laboratories have developed high-titer specific antibodies for individual neurophysins.

When neurophysins were originally isolated from the posterior pituitary, there was little hope that hormone-specific neurophysins could be identified. In several species several proteins were isolated, all of which had the ability to bind reversibly both vasopressin and oxytocin.[8-11] Subsequently, it was determined that many of the neurophysins in these extracts were degraded enzymatically in vitro. Using more careful extraction methods two major neurophysins were identified in most species.[12] When neurosecretory granules from bovine neurohypophyses were isolated by density gradient centrifugation, respective enrichment of granules containing bovine neurophysin I and oxytocin and of granules containing bovine neurophysin II and vasopressin was found.[13] This was the first evidence that one neurophysin was anatomically segregated with one hormone, a finding that has been amply confirmed by recent studies. The release of neurophysins was also originally demonstrated by biochemical techniques. Based on the anatomic studies of posterior pituitary secretion by Douglas,[14] which showed that the entire content of secretory granules left the cell by exocytosis, and the earlier demonstration that neurophysins are associated with the hormones within the granules, parallel secretion of the neurophysins was predicted. This hypothesis was proved by the work of Fawcett et al.,[15] who showed that a neurophysinlike peptide was released into the general circulation. These workers injected ^{35}S-labeled cysteine into the third ventricle of the dog. After sufficient time had elapsed to permit the cysteine to be incorporated into vasopressin, the dogs were subjected to hemorrhage to stimulate release of vasopressin, and radioactive materials were recovered from the peripheral blood. In addition to the finding of radioactive counts associated with vasopressin, counts were found in association with a 10,000-molecular-weight peptide, which was tentatively identified as neurophysin. In studies in the same laboratory by Sachs et al.,[16] it was shown that neurophysins were synthesized concurrently with vasopressin and that inhibition of synthesis of neurophysin always resulted in inhibition of synthesis of vasopressin. These workers hypothesized that neurophysin and vasopressin were synthesized as parts of a common precursor molecule.

Gainer (Chapter 3) has outlined the evidence that has confirmed the original hypothesis of Sachs et al. While these studies with biochemical techniques provided the initial support for the three areas of interest for neurophysins, the development of antibodies reactive with individual neurophysins made possible rapid advancement in each of the three areas of investigation.

2. CLASSIFICATION OF NEUROPHYSINS

In the original isolation of bovine and porcine neurophysins, the polypeptides were identified by numbers based on their electrophoretic mobility, the neurophysin moving most rapidly toward the anode being assigned the roman numeral I. This method has proven to be unsatisfactory because different laboratories have isolated different numbers of neurophysins. This was well demonstrated by reports of the isolation of human neurophysins in which one labortory identified two neurophysins and named them human neurophysins I and II,[17] whereas another laboratory identified four neurophysins in the human. Neurophysin III in the second laboratory was neurophysin I in the first laboratory.[18,19] There was also no correlation between the numbering system and the hormone with which the neurophysin was associated. Thus, bovine neurophysin I and porcine neurophysins II were each thought to be associated with oxytocin in their respective species.[19]

For biochemists who were determining the amino acid composition of neurophysins it was preferable to identify neurophysins based upon particular amino acids. Two classes of neurophysins were identified based on the amino acids in positions 2, 3, 6, and 7.[20,21] One class of neurophysins, designated MSEL, had Met, Ser, Glu, and Leu amino acids and the other, designated VLDV, had Val, Leu, Asp, and Val amino acids in the respective positions (Figure 1).

If it is correct that there is a hormone-specific neurophysin for vasopressin and one for oxytocin in each species, then the ideal classification would be to identify the vasopressin neurophysin and the oxytocin neurophysin in each species. One difficulty with this approach has been the identification of more than two neurophysins in several species. In four species in which more than two neurophysins have been identified, there is now good evidence that in each case the extra neurophysins are truncated forms of one of the two major neurophysins. In the cow[22] and in the human[18] there is complete antigenic

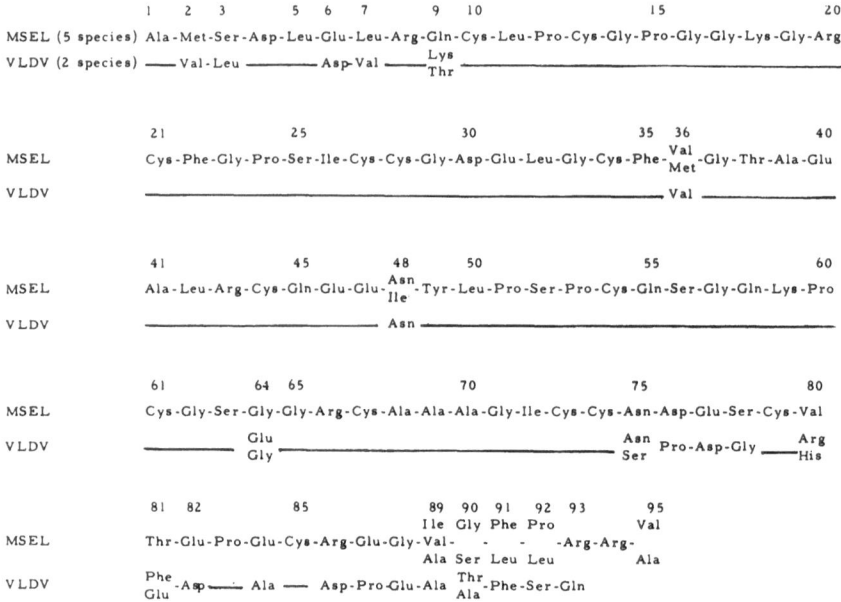

FIGURE 1. Comparison of two classes of neurophysins as determined by amino acid composition. The upper line shows the sequence of MSEL neurophysins and the lower line, the sequences of VLDV neurophysins. Solid lines indicate sequences that are identical between MSEL and VLDV neurophysins. Substitutions within each family are indicated. (From ref. 21.)

similarity between the respective extra neurophysins and one of the two major neurophysins. In the pig, the third porcine neurophysin has been shown to be just three amino acids longer than porcine neurophysin I,[23] and in the rat turnover studies using labeled neurophysins in vivo were consistent with the view that two neurophysins are synthesized initially and that enzymatic conversion takes place within the secretory granules of one of the two to form a third neurophysin.[24] In the human, partial amino acid sequencing has further proven that the two neurophysins that are antigenically similar are also identical in amino acid composition, with the exception of a few amino acids on the carboxy terminus[25] (similar to the description in the porcine neurophysins). Because extracts of fresh pituitary extracted very rapidly contain some of the extra neurophysins, it is apparent that there is intragranular breakdown of some of the neurophysins to produce neurophysin peptides with somewhat different biochemical characteristics. Perhaps the enzymes within the granule that cleave the neurophysin and the hormone from the common precursor molecule (as discussed previously) also further cleave the neurophysins to produce some heterogeneity of "mature" neurophysins.

It is clear from the foregoing discussion that biochemical classification of neurophysins alone has not identified the vasopressin neurophysin and the oxytocin neurophysin in given species. Three methods are available for such identification. When the common precursors are sequenced for each hormone in each species the hormone-specific neurophysin will be known. If specific antibodies are available for the individual neurophysins and the hormones vasopressin and oxytocin, then specific immunohistologic techniques should identify one neurophysin with one hormone in a given group of magnocellular neurons and the other neurophysin with the other hormone in a separate group of magnocellular neurons. Alternatively, if specific radioimmunoassays are available for each of the neurophysins and for each of the hormones, then with stimulated release of the hormone one might measure concurrent release of a specific neurophysin into the circulation to identify the hormone-specific neurophysin. There are four species in which anatomic and/or physiologic data have clearly identified hormone-specific neurophysins.

2.1. Bovine Hormone-Specific Neurophysins

Bovine neurophysins were the first neurophysins for which specific radioimmunoassays were available.[26] In the cow, stimuli that are known to cause the release of vasopressin (dehydration, hypertonic saline infusion, and hemorrhage)[27,28] have all been demonstrated to cause the release of bovine neurophysin II without the release of bovine neurophysin I (Figure 2). During milking, either by hand or by machine, there was selective release of bovine neurophysin I unaccompanied by release of bovine neurophysin II (Figure 3).[29]

2.2. Porcine Hormone-Specific Neurophysins

In the pig specific radioimmunoassays have been described by Dax et al.[30] Graded hemorrhage produced a 2- to 25-fold increase in porcine neurophysin I, while at parturition with the delivery of each piglet there was a 10-fold increase in porcine neurophysin II. Dehydration and suckling gave variable results in the pig.

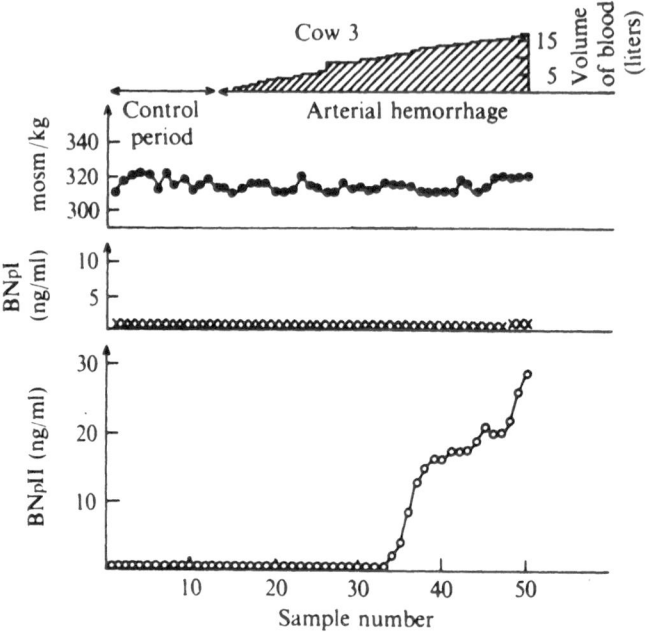

FIGURE 2. Release of bovine neurophysin II without concurrent release of bovine neurophysin I during continuous arterial hemorrhage in the cow. (From ref. 27.)

2.3. Rat Hormone-Specific Neurophysins

In the rat the most complete studies of release of neurophysin have utilized a homologous assay for rat neurophysin that did not distinguish between individual neurophysins.[31] There was, however, elevation in the level of neurophysin in plasma after injection of hypertonic saline, dehydration, hemorrhage, and also during parturition. It is in the Brattleboro rat that hormone-specific neurophysins have been proven. Brattleboro rats homozygous for diabetes insipidus lack vasopressin and lack one of the rat neurophysins, as identified by disc gel electrophoresis.[32]

2.4. Human Hormone-Specific Neurophysins

In the human a neurophysin designated as nicotine-stimulated neurophysin is now recognized as the vaospressin neurophysin of man.[18,19] Levels of this neurophysin in plasma increase in response to volume changes induced by tilt-table testing of normal human subjects and increase in response to osmotic stimulation produced by the standard Hicky–Hare test.[33] In studies of smoking in normal human volunteers there was an excellent correlation between the release of vasopressin and the release of nicotine-stimulated neurophysin (Figure 4), and prior administration of ethanol, which is known to block the release of vasopressin, inhibited the release of both vasopressin and nicotine-stimulated neurophysin in response to smoking.[34] The other neurophysin in the human has been designated estrogen-stimulated neuro-

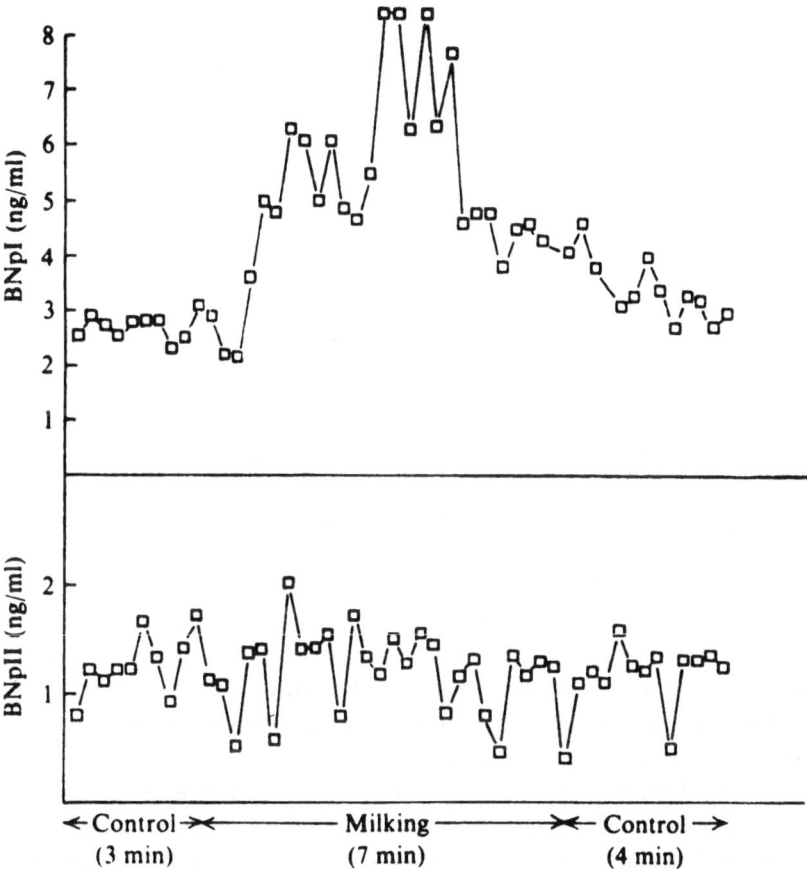

FIGURE 3. Release of bovine neurophysin I without release of bovine neurophysin II in the cow during hand-milking. (From ref. 29.)

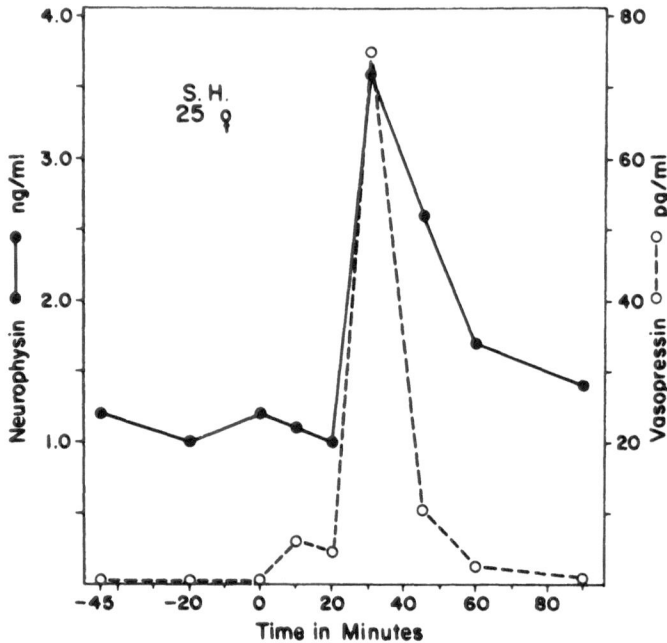

FIGURE 4. Levels of vasopressin neurophysin and of vasopressin in the human after smoking two cigarettes at 20 min. (From ref. 34.)

physin, and considerable data now support the hypothesis that this is the oxytocin neurophysin of man.[19] In studies of the human hypothalamus utilizing specific antineurophysin, immunostaining patterns associated the nicotine-stimulated neurophysins with the neurons that also contained vasopressin and the estrogen-stimulated neurophysin with the neurons that also contained oxytocin.[35] Recently the development of a radioimmunoassay for oxytocin has confirmed an excellent correlation between the chronic levels of oxytocin and of estrogen-stimulated neurophysin in women receiving estrogen-containing oral contraceptive tablets (Figure 5) and acute levels in normal subjects after taking a single tablet containing estrogen (Figure 6).[36] In more recent studies T. Herman, J. Stern, S. Reichlin, and A. G. Robinson have shown elevated levels of estrogen-stimulated neurophysin in normal women during breast-feeding and have correlated these levels with release of oxytocin (unpublished observations).

2.5. Stimulus-Specific Release of Individual Neurophysins

The correlation between the release of an individual hormone and that of an individual neurophysin has provided strong evidence to associate a given neurophysin with a given hormone in an individual species. However, the specific ability of the stimulus to release only one hormone of the posterior pituitary probably depends upon the strength of the stimulus applied and may vary greatly among species. For example, parturition is thought to be associated with the release of oxytocin, but in some women during parturition

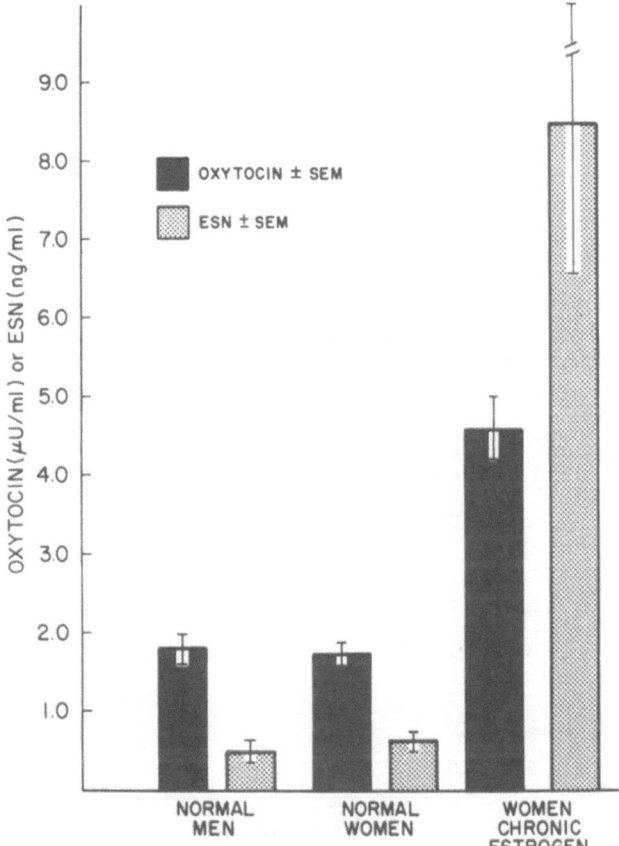

FIGURE 5. Levels of estrogen-stimulated neurophysin and of oxytocin in normal subjects and in women chronically taking oral contraceptive tablets. (From ref. 36.)

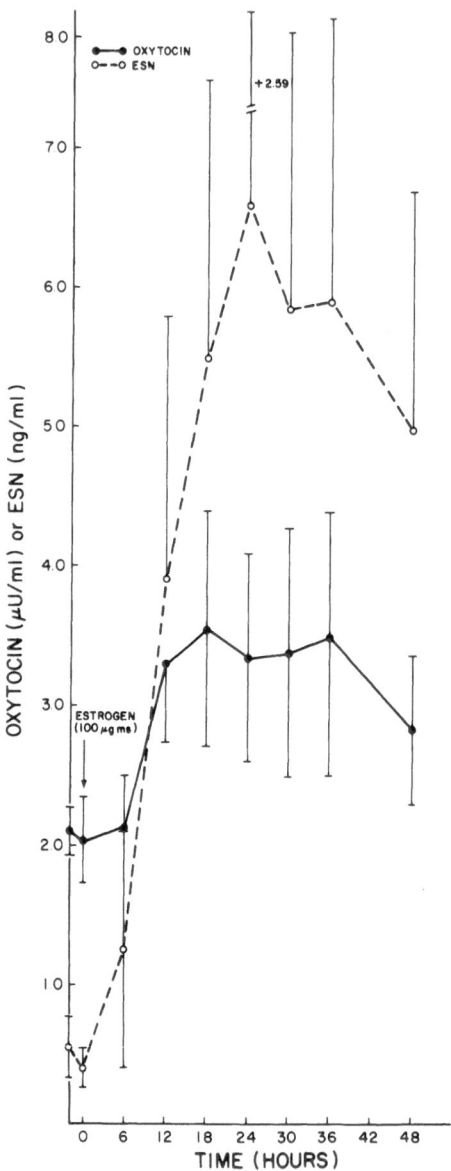

FIGURE 6. Levels of estrogen-stimulated neurophysin and of oxytocin in four subjects given 100 μg mestranol at time 0. Simultaneous release of oxytocin and estrogen-stimulated neurophysin was demonstrated. (From ref. 36.)

nicotine-stimulated neurophysin, the vasopressin neurophysin, was elevated.[33] In the cow vasopressin neurophysin was also elevated during the expulsive stage of labor.[29] In the rat we have clearly demonstrated an elevation of oxytocin in response to both administration of hypertonic saline (Figure 7) and hemorrhage. In fact, administration of hypertonic saline intraperitoneally to the rat results in a greater release of oxytocin than of vasopressin.[37]

2.6. Conclusions Regarding Classification of Neurophysins

The neurophysins that can be identified as vasopressin neurophysins by changes during appropriate stimulation—bovine neurophysin II, porcine neu-

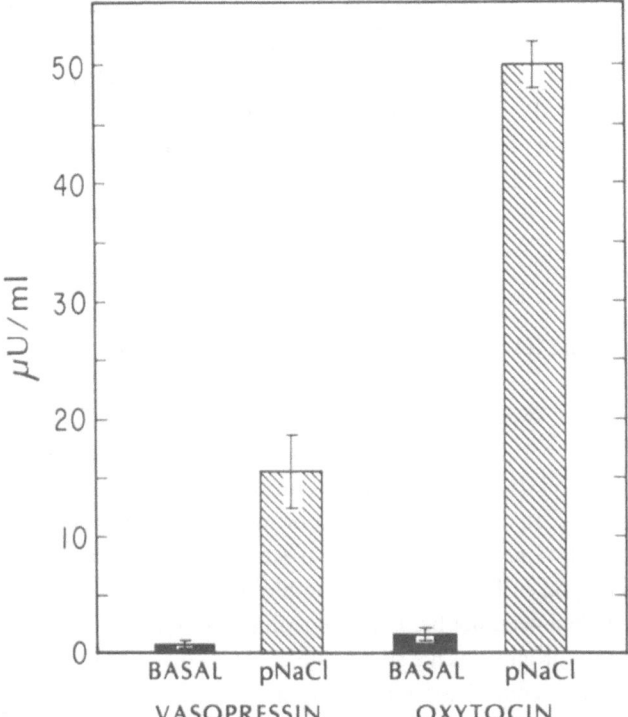

FIGURE 7. Overlap in stimulated release of oxytocin and of vasopressin in response to hypertonic saline in the rat. Three percent of body weight injected intraperitoneally as 5 g/100 ml NaCl; blood collected at 45 min. (From ref. 37.)

rophysin I, and human nicotine-stimulated neurophysin—have been identified as MSEL neurophysins based on amino acid composition. All of the neurophysins that have been identified as oxytocin neurophysins—bovine neurophysin I, porcine neurophysin II, and human estrogen-stimulated neurophysin—have been identified as VLDV neurophysins based on amino acid composition.[19] Thus, there may be specific amino acid sequence similarities between the hormone-specific neurophysins across species just as there are for the hormones themselves.

3. NEUROPHYSIN PATHWAYS AND SITES OF SECRETION

As described by Zimmerman and colleagues (Chapter 2), neurophysins have been proven by immunohistologic techniques to exist in association with the neurophypophysial hormones throughout the entire system of synthesis and secretion. With immunohistologic techniques it has been demonstrated that there are four sites of secretion of neurophysins: secretion from the posterior pituitary, secretion from the median eminence into the long portal vessels leading to the anterior pituitary, direct secretion into cerebrospinal fluid, and "ectopic" secretion by tumors.

3.1. Physiologic Secretion from the Posterior Pituitary

In all of the experiments described in which individual neurophysins were measured in peripheral blood at the time of stimulated release of oxytocin and/or of vasopressin, it is likely that the peptides were secreted by the posterior pituitary. In rats this can be documented by measurement of depletion of hormone and of neurophysin in the posterior pituitary concomitant with increased secretion of hormone and neurophysin into the peripheral blood.[31] Most of these data need not be reviewed at this time because for the secretion of vasopressin neurophysins the studies are confirmatory of physiologic factors that are known to control the release of vasopressin, i.e., vasopressin neurophysin is released in response to osmoreceptor and baroreceptor stimulation.[19] It need only be added that in many situations when the stimulus is mild there may be evidence of concentration of the urine or measured secretion of vasopressin that may not be accompanied by a measurable increase in the concentration of vasopressin neurophysin in plasma. This is probably due to the lack of sufficient sensitivity in the radioimmunoassays of human vasopressin neurophysin.[19]

With regard to the oxytocin neurophysin some new findings have emerged that may indicate heretofore unknown functions of oxytocin in the human. Prior to the identification of estrogen-stimulated neurophysin in the human, estrogen was not known to be a stimulus for the release of oxytocin. Yet, estrogen consistently stimulates the release of a specific neurophysin in the human and in the monkey.[33,38] This has been measured in response to pharmacologic doses of estrogen (as with oral contraceptive tablets), but also with physiologic changes in the level of estrogen in the circulation. Pregnancy in women is associated with an increase in this specific neurophysin from the second trimester through the duration of pregnancy.[33] In both women and monkeys the midcycle elevation of estrogen that is concurrent with the luteinizing hormone surge is associated with a midcycle elevation of estrogen-stimulated neurophysin[38] (Figure 8). Recent evidence in the human has confirmed that in each of these situations there is a concurrent increase in the level of oxytocin.[36,39] [Some preliminary studies in our laboratory indicate that detection of the elevated levels of oxytocin in response to administered estrogen depends upon the specific radioimmunoassay used. Some radioimmunoassays for oxytocin will detect this change in the level of oxytocin in plasma whereas other assays will not. Estrogens may not only stimulate the release of oxytocin and its respective neurophysin (estrogen-stimulated neurophysin) but also alter catabolism of oxytocin in plasma, so that one radioimmunoassay will recognize the metabolites whereas another radioimmunoassay may not.] The neurophysin, estrogen-stimulated neurophysin, is also elevated in pathologic states of estrogen excess, as in cirrhosis of the liver.[40]

3.2. Pathologic Secretion of Vasopressin

3.2.1. The Syndrome of Inappropriate Secretion of Antidiuretic Hormone

The syndrome of inappropriate secretion of antidiuretic hormone may occur because of release of vasopressin from the posterior pituitary or because of ectopic production and release of vasopressin by a tumor. In both situations

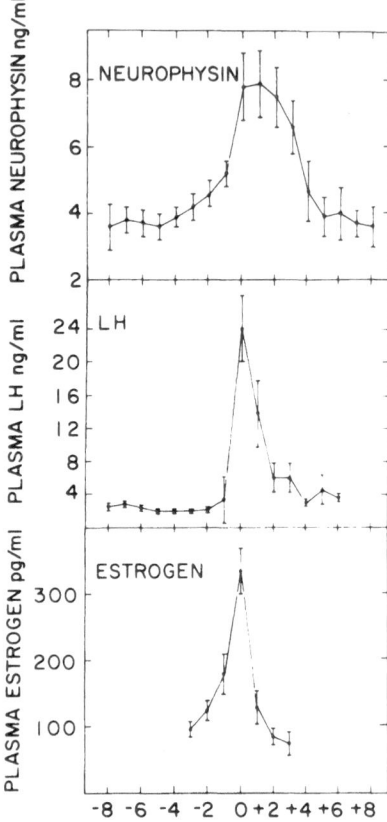

FIGURE 8. Levels of estrogen-stimulated neurophysin, luteinizing hormone, and estrogen in 19 monkeys at midcycle. The day of peak estrogen is represented by 0. (From ref. 38.)

elevated levels of neurophysin have been measured in plasma.[33,41] The highest levels occur in patients with lung cancer associated with production of vasopressin. Ectopic vasopressin neurophysin secretion is not influenced by usually appropriate physiologic stimuli. When tested with nicotine, water loading, or ingestion of alcohol, patients with cancer showed no change in plasma levels of neurophysin.[33] In studies by Yamaji et al., an oat cell carcinoma of the lung was maintained by continuous transplantation subcutaneously in the nude mouse.[42,43] Incubation of cell suspensions of this oat cell carcinoma with radiolabeled cysteine conclusively demonstrated the biosynthesis of neurophysins (along with vasopressin). North et al.[44] described the usefulness of measurement of human neurophysins as a tumor marker for oat cell carcinoma of the lung. In their study of 61 patients with small cell

carcinoma of the lung, 62% were found to have values of vasopressin neurophysin greater than three times normal. Furthermore there was good agree-
ment between changes in levels of neurophysin in plasma and the clinical
response of the patients to therapy (Figure 9). In some patients in whom there
was a lowering of the level of vasopressin neurophysin with antitumor therapy,
the neurophysin value became elevated again several weeks before it was
recognized that the patient was experiencing recurrence of the disease. In our
own series of 37 cases with oat cell carcinoma,[45] we also observed extraor-
dinarily high levels of nicotine-stimulated neurophysin, but did not find a

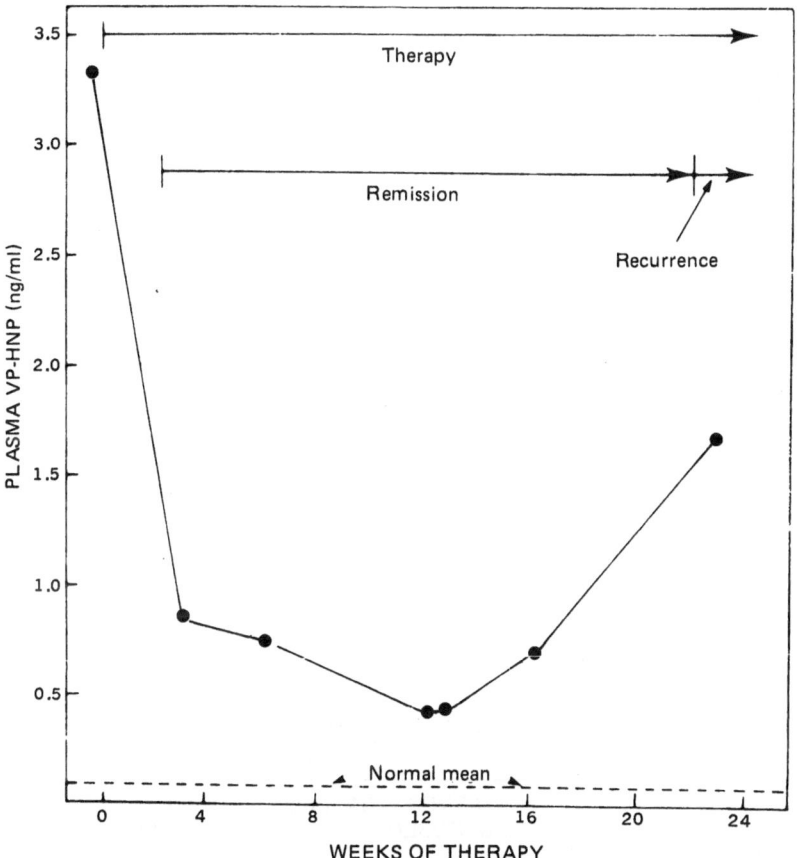

FIGURE 9. Levels of vasopressin neurophysin in man during therapy for oat cell carcinoma
associated with inappropriate secretion of antidiuretic hormone. Value of measured neurophysin
as index of response of tumor to therapy is noted. (From ref. 44.)

close correlation between the levels of neurophysin in plasma and clinical responsiveness. We also observed three patients in whom there was a marked increase in the level of neurophysin and no change in the level of vasopressin or an increase in the level of vasopressin without a corresponding elevation of neurophysin. It seems quite likely that in some cancers the precursor molecule may be cleaved in an abnormal manner so that some of the neurophysin or some of the vasopressin may not be detected by particular radioimmunoassays for these peptides. This possibility was well demonstrated by the oat cell carcinoma described by Pettengill et al.[46] When this tumor was grown in tissue culture, vasopressin was detected in media and localized by immunohistochemical techniques, but no neurophysin was demonstrated either in the media or in the tumor with radioimmunoassay and immunohistochemical techniques that had been amply verified as able to measure and detect neurophysin in other tissues in other experimental studies.

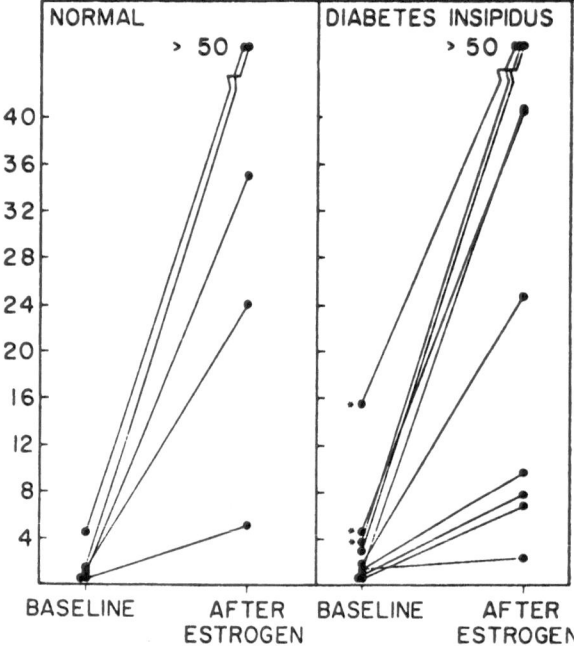

FIGURE 10. Estrogen-stimulated neurophysin in normal subjects (left) and patients with diabetes insipidus (right) before and after administration of estrogen. The "after" sample is the peak response to either 12, 24, or 36 hr. The starred samples are patients taking estrogen-containing oral contraceptives.

In some cancers there is elevation of the neurophysin associated with oxytocin, and it is likely that some tumors produce oxytocin ectopically.[33] There is no known pathologic disturbance associated with ectopic production of oxytocin, and the incidence of this disorder has not been described.

3.2.2. Diabetes Insipidus

As would be anticipated from the demonstrated deficiency of vasopressin in diabetes insipidus, its associated neurophysin is always lacking as well. On the other hand, virtually all patients with diabetes insipidus have responded with an elevation of the neurophysin associated with oxytocin (Figure 10). Intact oxytocin secretion was found in idiopathic diabetes insipidus and also in traumatic and postsurgical diabetes insipidus.[33] This was also noted in experimental diabetes insipidus produced by posterior lobe hypophysectomy in rats. In these rats the levels of vasopressin decreased from 1.7 to 0.5 pg/ml, consistent with diabetes insipidus, but the levels of oxytocin actually increased from 9 to 15 pg/ml.[47] Thus, the oxytocin system seems to be much less susceptible to damage than does the vasopressin-secreting system.[33] This may be the reason that many patients with diabetes insipidus have had relatively normal labor and delivery.

3.3. Secretion at the Median Eminence

It is of historic interest that Bargmann and Scharrer[48] in 1951 showed projections of neurohypophysial axons to the third ventricle and to the median eminence by histochemical studies using the Gomori stain. (Figure 11). Twenty years later the increased sensitivity provided by immunohistochemistry of neurophysins proved conclusively that neurophysin-containing axons terminate in the external zone of the median eminence.[49,50] Radioimmunoassays of blood obtained from the long portal vessels that drain from the median eminence to the anterior pituitary demonstrated concentrations of neurophysin and vasopressin in portal blood 50–400 times greater than those in simultaneously obtained samples of peripheral plasma.[51] The studies of Antunes et al.[52] have proven by unilateral lesions of the paraventricular nucleus that the projection of vasopressin neurons to the median eminence originates in the ipsilateral paraventricular nucleus. These studies are more completely described in Chapter 2.

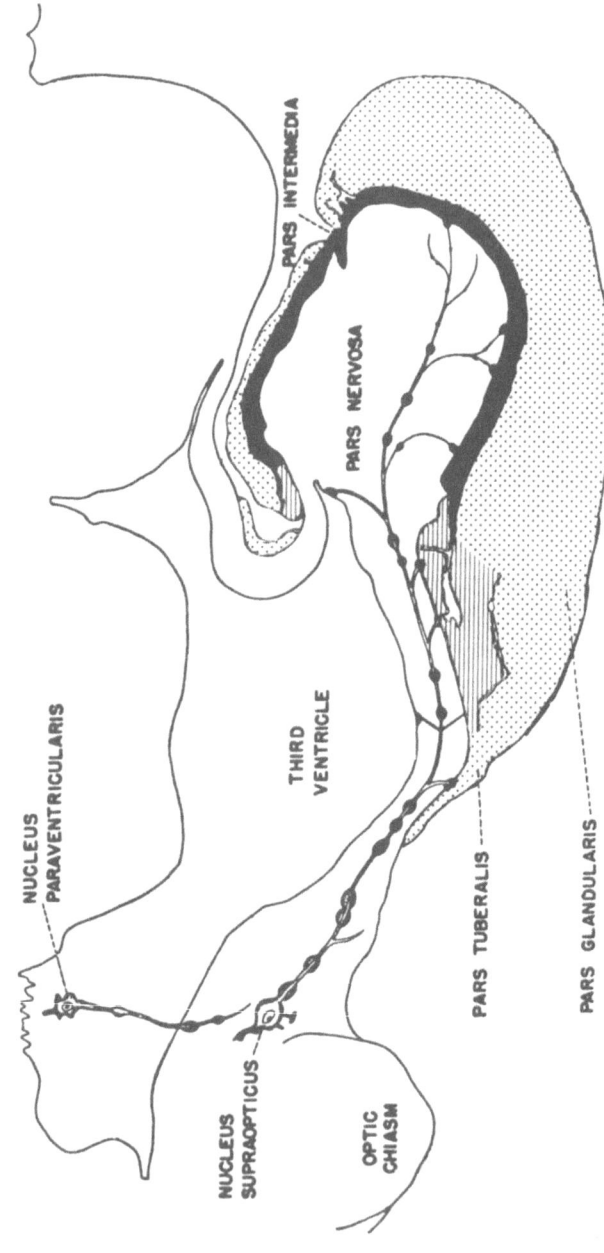

FIGURE 11. Supraopticohypophysial track as drawn by Bargmann and Scharrer in 1951. In addition to the axons to the pars nervosa, branches were drawn to the median eminence and to the infundibular recess of the third ventricle. (From ref. 48.)

It is well known that vasopressin can stimulate the release of adreno-corticotropic hormone (ACTH) but that there is another more potent corti-cotropin-releasing factor that is present in the hypothalamus.[53] What is not known is whether the secretion of vasopressin into the portal system influences the secretory activity of the anterior pituitary under physiological conditions. Many studies have confirmed that adrenalectomy is associated with an increase in neurophysin and vasopressin in the external zone, as determined both by immunohistochemical study of tissue sections[54–56] and by direct radioim-munoassay of biopsies of the external zone.[57] Dornhorst et al. studied the release of vasopressin and of ACTH in cats by placing electrodes in the paraventricular nucleus and the supraoptic nucleus and then measuring the concurrent release of ACTH and vasopressin after stimulation.[58] Stimulations in the region of the supraoptic nucleus resulted in release of vasopressin but no measured increase in the concentration of ACTH. In the paraventricular nucleus stimulation of most areas resulted in release of vasopressin and parallel release of ACTH, although in some areas there was release of ACTH without measured release of vasopressin (Figure 12). These data were consistent with the hypothesis that vasopressin was an intermediate to stimulate the release of ACTH, which was noted in response to stimulation of areas in the para-ventricular nucleus. The lack of measured elevation of vasopressin in con-currence with release of ACTH by stimulation of some other areas of the paraventricular nucleus may indicate that some areas in this nucleus make another corticotropin-releasing factor or that the release of vasopressin oc-curred only at the median eminence and that the magnitude of release was not sufficient to increase the concentration in the peripheral circulation.

Next, Carlson et al.[59] tested the possibility that blockade of vasopressin action after stimulation of the paraventricular nucleus would block the release of ACTH. Cats were treated as previously but stimulation of the paraven-tricular nucleus was performed in a basal state, after intraventricular injection of an antiserum against oxytocin, and after intraventricular injection of an antiserum against vasopressin. As in the initial study, stimulation of the paraventricular nucleus in control studies resulted in release of ACTH. This response was unaffected by intraventricular injection of hyperimmune rabbit serum or of antiserum directed against oxytocin, but when antiserum directed against vasopressin was injected intraventricularly, there was either complete blockade or a marked decrease in the release of ACTH. On the other hand stimulation of the anteroventral hypothalamus resulted in release of ACTH, which was not affected by intraventricular administration of antiserum to

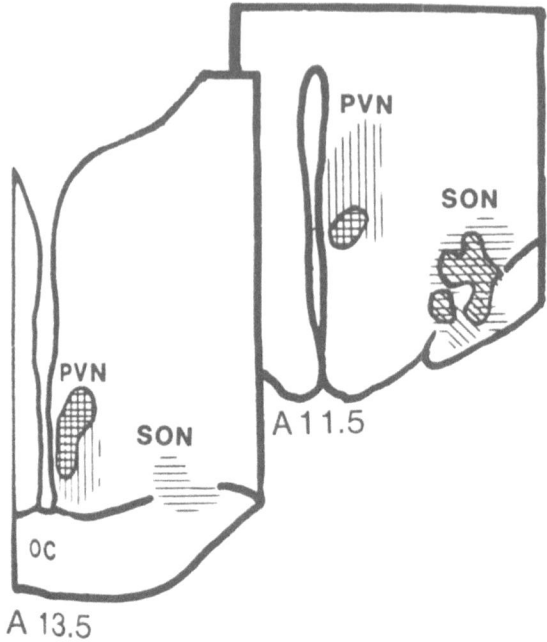

FIGURE 12. Release of ACTH and of vasopressin in response to stimulation of the paraventricular nucleus (PVN) and supraoptic nucleus (SON) of the cat. Vertical lines indicate areas in which stimulation facilitated release of ACTH. Horizontal lines indicate facilitation of release of vasopressin. Diagonal lines indicate inhibition of release of ACTH. Overlapping of vertical and of horizontal lines occurs only in the PVN. Stimulation of these areas resulted in simultaneous release of vasopressin and ACTH. (From ref. 58.)

vasopressin (Figure 13). The studies provide strong evidence that release of ACTH in response to stimulation of the paraventricular nucleus is via an intermediate release of vasopressin. The studies also prove that in other areas of the hypothalamus, e.g. the antroventral hypothalamus, release of ACTH is via some non-vasopressin corticotropin releasing activity. Vasopressin may be an intermediate for the release of ACTH in response to stimulation of the paraventricular nucleus, but the question of physiologic function of this pathway remains to be determined.

3.4. Secretion into Cerebrospinal Fluid

For many years vasopressin was known to be present in cerebrospinal fluid (CSF), but it was not established whether there was direct secretion of neurohypophysial peptides into the ventricular system.[60] Immunohistologic studies localized neurophysins close to the base of the third ventricle in a position that suggested that there could be secretion of neurophysins into the ventricular system.[61,62] When neurophysins were measured in CSF of monkey and man the levels were found to be higher than levels in peripheral blood.[63] The possibility has been considered that neurophysins enter the CSF from peripheral blood. In earlier studies, seven dogs were injected with bovine neurophysin, which could be specifically measured without interference with the natural neurophysin present in the dog.[63] Although high concentrations of neurophysin were present in the peripheral plasma, there was no transfer

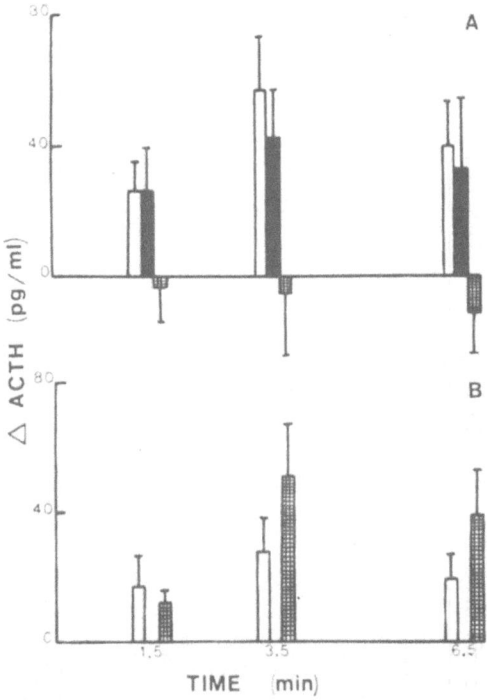

FIGURE 13. Release of ACTH 1.5, 3.5, and 6.5 min after stimulation of the paraventricular nucleus (A) and of the anteroventral hypothalamus (B). Open bars are control stimulation and demonstrate increased release of ACTH. Solid bars are stimulation after intraventricular administration of hyperimmune serum or antiserum to oxytocin and demonstrate no change in release of ACTH in the top graph. Cross-hatched bars demonstrate stimulated release of ACTH after intraventricular administration of antiserum to vasopressin. In the PVN there was decreased stimulation of ACTH after administration of antiserum to vasopressin. In the anteroventral hypothalamus there was no change. (From ref. 59.)

TABLE I. Effect of Intravenous Bovine Neurophysin on Plasma and CSF Neurophysin Concentrations in Dogs[a]

	Dog 1		Dog 2		Dog 3		Dog 4		Dog 5		Dog 6		Dog 7		Dog 8	
	Plasma	CSF	Plasma	CSF	Plasma	CSF	Plasma	CSF	Plasma	CSF	Plasma	CSF	Plasma	CSF	Plasma	CSF
−60 min	<0.4		<0.4		<0.4		<0.4		<0.4		<0.4		<0.4		<0.4	
−40 min	<0.4		<0.4		<0.4		<0.4		<0.4		<0.4		<0.4		<0.4	
−20 min	<0.4		<0.4		<0.4		<0.4		<0.4		<0.4		<0.4		<0.4	
0 min																
2 min	115.0		122.0		63.0		103.0		105.0		65.0		37.0		28.0	
5 min	79.0		48.0		35.0		54.0		67.0		39.0		18.0		12.0	
15 min	25.0		35.0		16.0		21.0		20.0		14.0		7.0		4.0	
30 min	14.0		10.8		5.2		16.4		17.6		6.0	<0.4	3.0	0.5		<0.4
45 min	5.0	5.0	0.5		0.6	<0.4	1.2		4.0		3.8		1.4		1.2	
75 min	0.8				0.6		1.0	<0.4	1.8	0.5	1.6		0.8		0.6	<0.4
105 min	0.4	<0.4									1.2		0.7			<0.4

[a] Intravenous injection of bovine neurophysin into eight dogs. Dogs 1–5 received 375 μg of crude bovine neurophysin. Dog 6 received 100 μg of purified bovine neurophysin I, and dogs 7 and 8 received 50 μg of purified bovine neurophysin I. Bovine neurophysin I was determined by radioimmunoassay on samples of plasma and CSF.[63]

of neurophysin from the plasma to the cerebroventricular system, as documented by serial measurements of CSF (Table I). Taken together the studies indicate that the high levels of neurophysin detected in the CSF of man and monkey were the result of direct secretion. Hypophysectomy in the rat decreased the levels of vasopressin in plasma from 1.7 to 0.5 pg/ml, while there was a simultaneous increase in the levels of vasopressin in the CSF from 12 to 37 pg/ml.[47] As described earlier, the levels of oxytocin increased in the plasma after hypophysectomy from 9 to 15 pg/ml, but the levels in the CSF were unchanged at 73 and 83 pg/ml. As hypophysectomy virtually eliminated the secretion of vasopressin into the peripheral plasma but not the levels in the CSF, the vasopressin that was released into the CSF apparently was released via a pathway independent of the pathway to the posterior pituitary lobe. That the levels of vasopressin in the CSF actually increased after hypophysectomy might indicate that secretion into the ventricular pathway in-

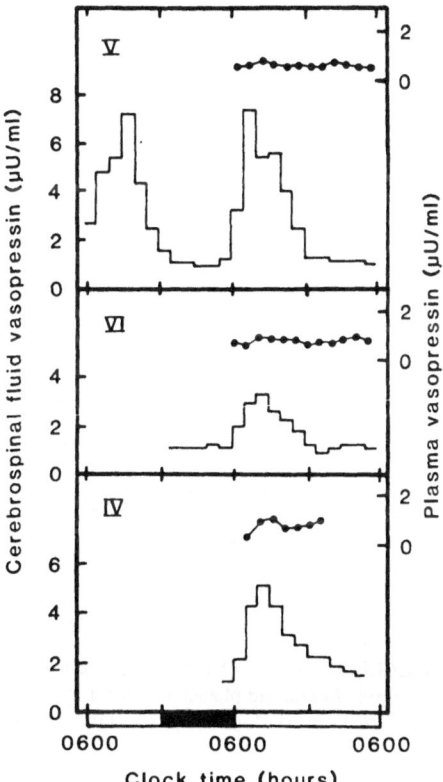

FIGURE 14. Pattern of vasopressin in CSF (bar graph) and plasma (closed circles) in three cats over a 24-hr period of constant light. Note no change in the levels of vasopressin in plasma but striking diurnal variation of vasopressin levels in CSF. (From ref. 64.)

creased in response to the diabetes insipidus caused by lack of vasopressin in the periphery.

Further evidence for the independence of the release of neurohypophysial peptides into CSF as compared to the peripheral plasma came from studies of the diurnal rhythm of vasopressin and oxytocin in CSF as compared with peripheral plasma. Reppert et al.[64] collected cisteral CSF continuously from adult male cats and measured the level of vasopressin in two-hourly samples. In each of five cats there was a marked diurnal pattern of vasopressin release, with a maximum of 4–7.5 μU/ml by 6–8 hr after light and a minimum shortly after the onset of darkness. The pattern persisted for three days of continuous light, indicating that the vasopressin rhythm was endogenously generated. It is important to emphasize that no rhythm of vasopressin could be shown in samples obtained from plasma of the same cats (Figure 14). Thus the concentrations of vasopressin detected in the CSF probably were secreted by a different group of neurons than those responsible for secretion of vasopressin into the peripheral blood. In similar studies Perlow et al.[65] obtained continuous samples of CSF from monkeys. In two-hourly samples there was a marked

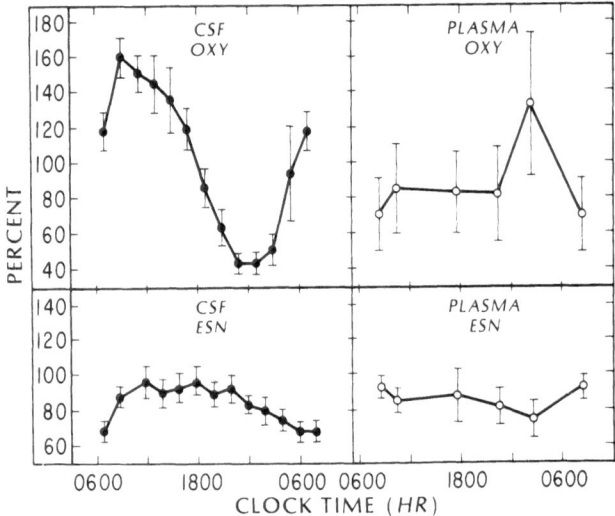

FIGURE 15. Levels of oxytocin and estrogen-stimulated neurophysin in CSF of four male monkeys. Results are plotted as percent increase or decrease from daily mean during the 24-hr day. Means ± SEM are indicated. (From ref. 65.)

rhythm of oxytocin and of the oxytocin neurophysin in the monkey (Figure 15). Daytime values of oxytocin in spinal fluid were 3- to 12-fold higher than nighttime values, with the nadir in the middle of the dark period and the peak early in the light period. The range of oxytocin in CSF was 5.2–10.2 μU/ml, significantly higher than simultaneously obtained levels in the peripheral blood. As with the levels of vasopressin in the cat, a daily rhythm of oxytocin in samples of plasma was not demonstrable. There was a rhythm of vasopressin in the CSF of the monkey, but the daily values were only twofold higher than nighttime values. Therefore the excursions of CSF vasopressin in the monkey were smaller than those in the cat and smaller than the rhythm of oxytocin in the monkey. Administration of estradiol benzoate dramatically increased the concentrations of estrogen-stimulated neurophysin in plasma for 4–5 days but did not alter the levels of oxytocin or of estrogen-stimulated neurophysin in CSF. As in the cat, the data offer convincing evidence that the axonal projections to the ventricular system function differently than the projections to the posterior pituitary.

There are different populations of oxytocin- and vasopressin-producing neurons within the hypothalamus with regard to both projections to the ventricular system and projections to the median eminence. It is probable that the different populations of neurons are indicative of different physiologic functions of the hormones. It is well known from studies in animals that injection of vasopressin into the ventricular system can cause changes in memory consolidation.[66] The finding of rhythmic secretion of neurohypophysial peptides into CSF increases the possibility that a function for these peptides in the brain distinct from the effects in the periphery will be discovered.

ACKNOWLEDGMENTS. Work reported herein was supported by NIH Grant AM 16166 and Clinical Research Grant RR-00056. I would like to thank Jane Pennebaker and Monica Rentz for secretarial support and Darinka Sipula and Ludka Stolc for laboratory assistance.

REFERENCES

1. Van Dyke HB, Chow BF, Greep RO, et al: The isolation of a protein from the pars neuralis of the ox pituitary with constant oxytocin, pressor and diuresis-inhibiting activities. *J Pharmacol Exp Ther* 74:190–209, 1942.

2. Van Dyke HB: Studies in neurohypophysial endocrinology. The Sir Henry Dale Lecture, 1970. *Proceedings of the Society of Endocrinology.* Meeting House, Zoological Society of London, 1970, pp x–xix.

3. Acher R, Chauvet J, Olivry O: Sur l'existence éventuelle d'une hormone unique neurohypophysaire. *Biochim Biophys Acta* 22:421–427, 1956.

4. Chauvet M, Chauvet J, Acher R: Phylogeny of neurophysins: Partial amino acid sequence of a sheep neurophysin. *FEBS Lett* 52:212–215, 1975.

5. Acher R, Chauvet J, Olivry G: Sur l'existence d'une hormone unique neurohypophysaire: Relation entre l'oxytocin, la vasopressine, et la protein de vanDyke extradites de la neurohypophyse du boeuf. *Biochem Biophys Acta* 22:428–433, 1956.

6. Sawyer WH: Evolution of antidiuretic hormones and their functions. *Am J Med* 42:678–691, 1967.

7. Heller H: History of neurohypophysial research, in Knobil E, Sawyer WH (eds): *Handbook of Physiology.* Baltimore, Waverly Press, 1974, vol 4, pp 103–117.

8. Hollenberg MD, Hope DB: Fractionation of neurophysin by molecular-sieve and ion-exchange chromatography. *Biochem J* 104:122–127, 1967.

9. DeMey J, Vandesande F, Dierickx K: Immunohistochemical identification of the neurophysin I and of the neurophysin II producing neurons in the bovine hypothalamus. *Ann Endocrinol (Paris)* 36:377–378, 1975.

10. Cheng KW, Friesen HG: Isolation and characterization of a third component of porcine neurophysin. *J Biol Chem* 246:7656–7665, 1971.

11. Uttenthal LO, Hope DB: The isolation of three neurophysins from porcine posterior lobes. *Biochem J* 116:899–909, 1970.

12. Hope DB: The neurophysin proteins: Historical aspects. *Ann NY Acad Sci* 248:6–14, 1975.

13. Dean CR, Hope DB, Kazic T: Evidence for a storage of oxytocin with neurophysin-I and of vasopressin with neurophysin-II in separate neurosecretory granules. *Br J Pharmacol* 34:192P-193P, 1968.

14. Douglas WW: Mechanism of release of neurohypophysial hormones: Stimulus secretion coupling, in Knobil E, Sawyer WH (eds): *Handbook of Physiology.* Baltimore, Waverly Press, 1974, vol 4, pp 191–224.

15. Fawcett CP, Powell AE, Sachs H: Biosynthesis and release of neurophysin. *Endocrinology* 83:1299–1310, 1968.

16. Sachs H, Fawcett P, Takabatake Y, et al: Biosynthesis and release of vasopressin and neurophysin. *Rec Prog Horm Res* 25:447–491, 1969.

17. Cheng KW, Friesen HG: Studies of human neurophysin by radioimmunoassay. *J Clin Endocrinol Metab* 34:165–176, 1972.

18. Robinson AG: Isolation assay and secretion of individual human neurophysins. *J Clin Invest* 55:360–367, 1975.

19. Robinson AG, Verbalis JG, Amico JA, et al: Recent advances in neurohypophyseal research, in McCann SM (ed): *International Review of Physiology.* Baltimore, University Park Press, vol 24, 1981.

20. Acher R, Chauvet J, Olivry G: The actual existence of a single pituitary hormone. I. Relation between the oxytocin, vasopressin, and Van Dyke's protein extracted from bovine pituitary. *Biochim Biophys Acta* 22:421–427, 1956.

21. Chauvet MT, Codogno R, Chauvet J, et al: Comparison between MSEL- and VLDV-neurophysins: Complete amino acid sequences of porcine and bovine VLDV-neurophysins. *FEBS Lett* 98:37–40, 1979.

22. DeMey J, Vandensande F: Bovine neurophysins I, II and C: New Methods for their purification and for the production of specific antibodies. *Eur J Biochem* 69:153–162, 1976.

23. Wuu T, Crumm SE: Characterization of porcine neurophysin III. Its resemblance and possible relationship to porcine neurophysin I. *J Biol Chem* 251:2735–2739, 1976.

24. Burford GD, Pickering BT: Intra-axonal transport and turnover of neurophysin in the rat: A proposal for a possible origin of the minor neurophysin component. *Biochem J* 136:1047–1052, 1973.

25. Chauvet MT, Chauvet J, Acher R, et al: Identification of MSEL- and VLDV-neurophysins in human pituitary gland. *FEBS Lett* 101:391–394, 1979.

26. Robinson AG, Zimmerman EA, Engleman EG, et al: Radioimmunoassay of bovine neurophysin: Specificity of neurophysin I and II. *Metabolism* 20:1138–1147, 1971.

27. Legros JJ, Reynaert R, Peeters G: Specific release of bovine neurophysin II during arterial or venous haemorrhage in the cow. *J Endocrinol* 67:297–302, 1975.

28. Robinson AG, Zimmerman EA, Frantz AG: Physiologic investigation of the posterior pituitary binding proteins neurophysin I and neurophysin II. *Metabolism* 20:1148–1155, 1971.

29. Legros JJ, Reynaert R, Peeters G: Specific release of bovine neurophysin I during milking and suckling in the cow. *J Endocrinol* 60:327–332, 1974.

30. Dax EM, Cumming IA, Lawson RAS, et al: The physiological release of specific individual neurophysins into the circulation in pigs. *Endocrinology* 100:635–641, 1977.

31. Seif SM, Huellmantel AB, Platia MP, et al: Isolation radioimmunoassay and physiologic secretion of rat neurophysins. *Endocrinology* 100:1317–1326, 1977.

32. Sunde DA, Sokol HW: Quantification of rat neurophysin by polyacrylamide gel electrophoresis (PAGE): Application to the rat with hereditary hypothalamic diabetes insipidus. *Ann NY Acad Sci* 248:345–364, 1975.

33. Robinson AG, Haluscczak C, Wilkins JA, et al: Physiologic control of two neurophysins in humans. *J Clin Endocrinol Metab* 44:330–339, 1977.

34. Husain MK, Frantz AG, Ciarochi FF, et al: Nicotine stimulated release of neurophysin and vasopressin in humans. *J Clin Endocrinol Metab* 41:1113–1117, 1975.

35. Zimmerman EA, Defendini R, Sokol HW, et al: The distribution of neurophysin-secreting pathways in the mammalian brain: Light microscopic studies using the immunoperoxidase technique. *Ann NY Acad Sci* 248:92–111, 1975.

36. Amico JA, Seif SM, Robinson AG: Oxytocin in human plasma: Correlation with neurophysin and stimulation with estrogen. *J Clin Endocrinol Metab* 52:988–993, 1981.

37. Seif SM, Huellmantel AB, Verbalis J, et al: Radioimmunoassay and physiological response of oxytocin in the rat. Personal communication.

38. Robinson AG, Ferin M, Zimmerman EA: Neurophysin secretion in monkeys: Emphasis on the hypothalamic response to estrogen and ovarian events. *Endocrinology* 98:468–475, 1976.

39. Amico JA, Seif SM, Robinson AG: Elevation of oxytocin and the oxytocin-associated neurophysin in the plasma of normal women during midcycle. *J Clin Endocrinol Metab* 53:1229–1232, 1981.

40. VanThiel DH, Gavaler JS, Lester R, et al: Plasma, estrone, prolactin, neurophysin, and sex steroid-binding globulin in chronic alcoholic men. *Metabolism* 24:1015–1019, 1975.

41. Hamilton BPM, Upton GV, Amatruda TT Jr: Evidence for the presence of neurophysin in tumors producing the syndrome of inappropriate antidiuresis. *J Clin Endocrinol Metab* 35:764–767, 1972.

42. Yamaji T, Ishibashi M, Katayama S: Nature of the immunoreactive neurophysins in ectopic vasopressin-producing oat cell carcinomas of the lung. *J Clin Invest* 68:388–398, 1981.

43. Yamaji T, Ishibashi M, Katayama S, et al: Neurophysin biosynthesis in vitro in oat cell carinoma of the lung with ectopic vasopressin production. *J Clin Invest* 68:1441–1449, 1981.

44. North WG, Maurer LH, Valtin H, et al: Human neurophysins as potential tumor markers for small cell carcinoma of the lung: Application of specific radioimmunoassays. *J Clin Endocrinol Metab* 51:892–896, 1980.
45. Parveen G, Robinson AG, Seif S, et al: Vasopressin and neurophysin in cancer. *Clin Res* 29(2):Abstract #298A, 1981.
46. Pettengill OS, Faulkner CS, Wurster-Hill DH, et al: Isolation and characterization of a hormone producing cell line from human cell anaplastic carcinoma of the lung. *J Natl Cancer Inst* 58:511–518, 1977.
47. Dogterom J, Van Wimersma Griednaus TJB, Swaab DF: Evidence for the release of vasopressin and oxytocin into cerebrospinal fluid: Measurements in plasma and CSF of intact and hypophysectomized rats. *Neuroendocrinology* 24:108–118, 1977.
48. Bargmann W, Scharrer E: The site of origin of the hormones of the posterior pituitary. *Am Sci* 39:255–259, 1951.
49. Zimmerman EA: Localization of hypothalamic hormones by immunocytochemical techniques, in Martini L, Ganong WF (eds): *Frontiers in Neuroendocrinology*. New York, Raven Press, 1976, vol 4, pp 25–62.
50. Stillman MA, Recht LD, Rosario SL, et al: The effects of adrenalectomy and glucocorticoid replacement on vasopressin and vasopressin–neurophysin in the zona externa of the median eminence of the rat. *Endocrinology* 101:42–49, 1977.
51. Zimmerman EA, Carmel PW, Husain MK, et al: Vasopressin and neurophysin: High concentrations in monkey hypophyseal portal blood. *Science* 182:925–927, 1973.
52. Antunes JL, Carmel PW, Zimmerman EA: Projections from the paraventricular nucleus to the zona externa of the median eminence of the rhesus monkey: An immunohistochemical study. *Brain Res* 131:1–10, 1977.
53. Sinding C, Robinson AG: Progress in endocrinology and metabolism: A review of neurophysins. *Metabolism* 26:1355–1370, 1977.
54. Dierickx K, Vandensande F, DeMey J: Identification and origin of the vasopressin–neurophysin containing nerve fibres of the external region of the rat median eminence. *Ann Endocrinol (Paris)* 36:383–384, 1975.
55. Schwabedal P, Bock R: Influence of adrenalectomy, total body X-irradiation and dexamethasone on the amount of CRF-granules and "classical" neurosecretory material in the rat neurohypophysis. *Anat Embryol* 148:267–278, 1975.
56. Watkins WB, Schwabedal P, Bock R: Immunohistochemical demonstration of a CRF-associated neurophysin in the external zone of the rat median eminence. *Cell Tissue Res* 152:411–421, 1974.
57. Seif SM, Robinson AG, Zimmerman EA, et al: Stimulated neurohypophyseal function after adrenalectomy. Fifth International Congress of Endocrinology, Hamburg, Germany, Abstract #179, July 22–24, 1976.
58. Dornhorst A, Carlson DE, Seif SM, et al: Control of release of adrenocorticotropin and vasopressin by the supraoptic and paraventricular nuclei. *Endocrinology* 108:1420–1424, 1981.
59. Carlson DE, Dornhorst A, Seif SM, et al: Vasopressin-dependent and -independent control of the release of adrenocorticotropin. *Endocrinology* 110:680–682, 1982.
60. Van Dyke HB: *The Physiology and Pharmacology of the Pituitary Body*. Chicago, University of Chicago Press, 1936, vol 1, p 333.
61. Scott DE, Kozlowski GP, Sheridan MN: Scanning electromicroscopy in the ultrastructural analysis of the mammalian cerebral ventricular system. *Int Rev Cytol* 37:349–388, 1974.
62. Defendini R, Zimmerman EA: The magnocellular neurosecretory system of the mammalian hypothalamus, in Reichlin S, Baldessarini RJ, Martin JB (eds): *The Hypothalamus*, New York, Raven Press, 1978, pp 137–154.

63. Robinson AG, Zimmerman EA: Cerebrospinal fluid and ependymal neurophysin. *J Clin Invest* 52:1260–1267, 1973.
64. Reppert SM, Artman HG, Swaminathan S, et al: Vasopressin exhibits a rhythmic daily pattern in cerebrospinal fluid but not in blood. *Science* 213:1256–1257, 1981.
65. Perlow MJ, Reppert SM, Artman HG, et al: Oxytocin, vasopressin and estrogen stimulated neurophysin: Daily patterns of concentration in cerebrospinal fluid. *Science* 216:1416–1418, 1982.
66. DeWied D: Hormonal influences on motivation, learning, memory and psychosis, in Krieger DT, Hughes KC (eds): *Neuroendocrinology*. Sunderland, Sinauer Associates, 1980, pp 194–204.

6

PATHOLOGY OF THE NEUROHYPOPHYSIS

Kalman Kovacs

This chapter deals with the conventional pathology of the human neurohy-pophysis and includes no details related to neurosecretion or correlations between neurohypophysial and adenohypophysial endocrine activity.

1. ANATOMY AND HISTOLOGY

Anatomically, the neurohypophysis consists of three parts: (1) the median eminence, (2) the infundibular stem or distal pituitary stalk, and (3) the posterior or neural lobe or infundibular process. The former two parts constitute the infundibulum or neural stalk and form the funnel-shaped upward extension of the pituitary; they will be discussed only briefly here. The latter part is located within the sella turcica, in close approximation to the anterior lobe, and is the principal subject of this chapter.

Although these three anatomic divisions represent a functional unit, they have different roles in the maintenance of endocrine homeostasis. The median eminence contains high concentrations of various releasing as well as inhibitory hormones and factors. Synthesized in different areas of the hypothalamus, these substances are transported from their production sites to the median eminence, and via the portal circulation to the anterior lobe.[1-3] The pituitary stalk has both a vascular and a neural component. The vascular component is comprised of the portal vessels, which carry blood from the median em-

Kalman Kovacs • Department of Pathology, St. Michael's Hospital, and University of Toronto, Toronto, Ontario M5B 1W8, Canada.

inence region to the anterior lobe. The portal circulation not only supplies oxygen and other nutrients to the anterior pituitary but also transports hypothalamic hormones and factors, hence its integrity is of fundamental importance in the regulation of adenohypophysial endocrine activity. The neural component consists of the unmyelinated nerve fibers of the supraopticohypophysial and tuberohypophysial tracts. The former originates in the supraoptic and paraventricular nuclei, the latter in the middle and posterior hypothalamus. The supraoptic and paraventricular nuclei, the magnocellular nuclei of the hypothalamus, are located in the anterior hypothalamus and are the production sites of vasopressin and oxytocin. These two posterior pituitary hormones, bound to their carrier proteins, neurophysins, are transported along the nerve fibers of the supraopticohypophysial tract by axonal flow via the pituitary stalk to the posterior lobe; they are stored at the nerve endings of the posterior lobe and released into the circulation.[1,4] The axons contain actin filaments, suggesting that contractile proteins may be involved in the axonal transport of neurosecretory material and in hormone discharge.[5]

The posterior lobe is the downward extension of the central nervous system into the sella turcica. Unlike the anterior lobe, which is assumed to derive from Rathke's pouch, it originates from the floor of the diencephalon, the so-called saccus infundibularis. It is well developed and contains both vasopressin and oxytocin at birth.[6] The neurosecretory material is easily recognizable at approximately 5 months of intrauterine life, and it is abundant at the end of pregnancy.[7,8]

Grossly, the grayish posterior lobe is sharply demarcated from the reddish-brown anterior lobe. It is smaller than the anterior lobe; it comprises approximately 20% of the entire organ and weighs approximately 0.10–0.15 g.

Histologically, the posterior lobe is composed of nerve fibers, axon terminals, pituicytes, and neurosecretory material, which corresponds to vasopressin, oxytocin, and neurophysins (Figure 1). The neurosecretory granules can be demonstrated histologically in the posterior lobe, stalk, median eminence, and appropriate areas of the hypothalamus by various staining methods, such as Gomori's chromalum–hematoxylin, aldehyde–fuchsin, or aldehyde–thionin stains and, at the light and electron microscopic levels, by the reliable, sensitive, and specific immunoperoxidase technique.[9–13] The ultrastructural features of the infundibulum, stalk, and posterior lobe have been described in detail[14–20] (Figures 2–4).

The posterior lobe has a rich vascular supply thought to be independent of the anterior lobe. The inferior hypophysial arteries, branches of the internal

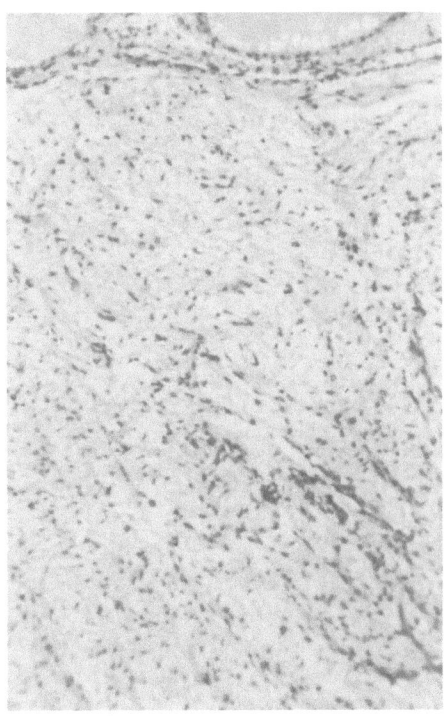

FIGURE 1. Histologic appearance of the posterior lobe. Hematoxylin–phloxin–saffron. Magnification 100 × .

carotid arteries, provide blood to the posterior lobe. The superior hypophysial arteries supply the anterior lobe. Capillaries within the posterior and anterior lobes are lined by fenestrated endothelium. Recent evidence seems to indicate that the neurohypophysis plays an important role in the regulation of circulation in the pituitary–median eminence area.[21] Blood from the posterior lobe can flow to the systemic circulation by way of the anterior lobe, in that the short portal vessels originate in the posterior lobe and terminate in the adenohypophysis. Under certain conditions, blood flow may be reversed, circulating from the adenohypophysis to the posterior lobe, and from there via the pituitary stalk to the median eminence. These findings, if sufficiently confirmed, will be important from the functional point of view, as they provide the anatomical basis for transport of various endocrinologically active substances from the anterior lobe to the posterior lobe and to the hypothalamus.[22]

The posterior lobe has a rich, direct nerve supply and is in close anatomic and functional contact with the hypothalamus. As discussed previously, two tracts—the supraopticohypophysial and the tuberohypophysial—connect the hypothalamus with the posterior lobe.

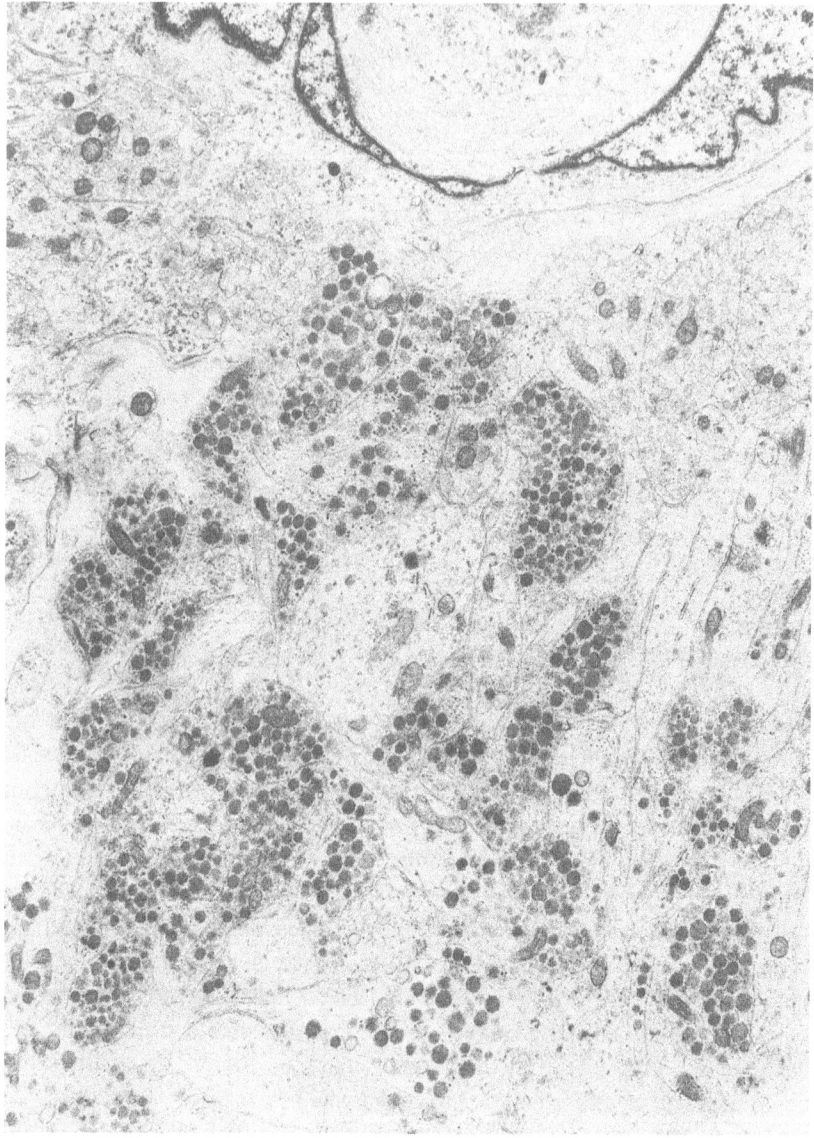

FIGURE 2. Electron micrograph of the posterior lobe showing nerve fibers containing neurosecretory granules. 10,000 × .

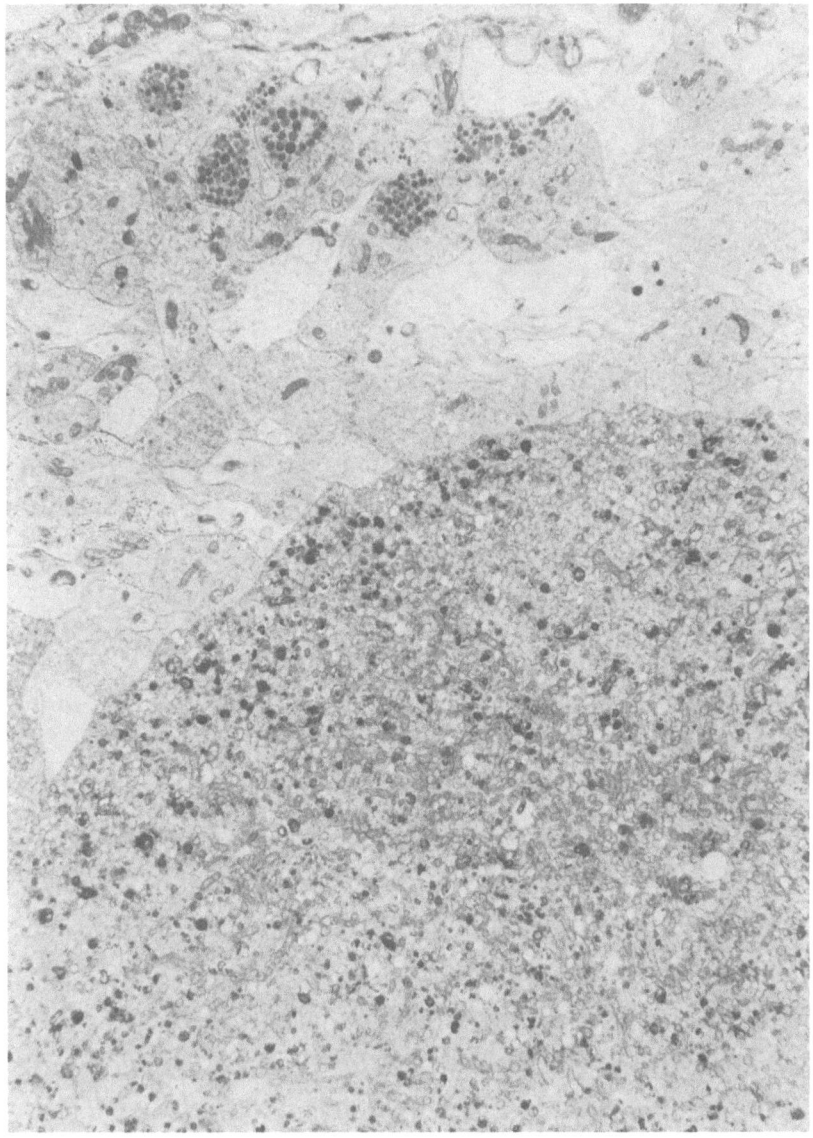

FIGURE 3. Electron micrograph of the posterior lobe showing a focally dilated axon terminal filled with neurosecretory material (Herring body). 5700 × .

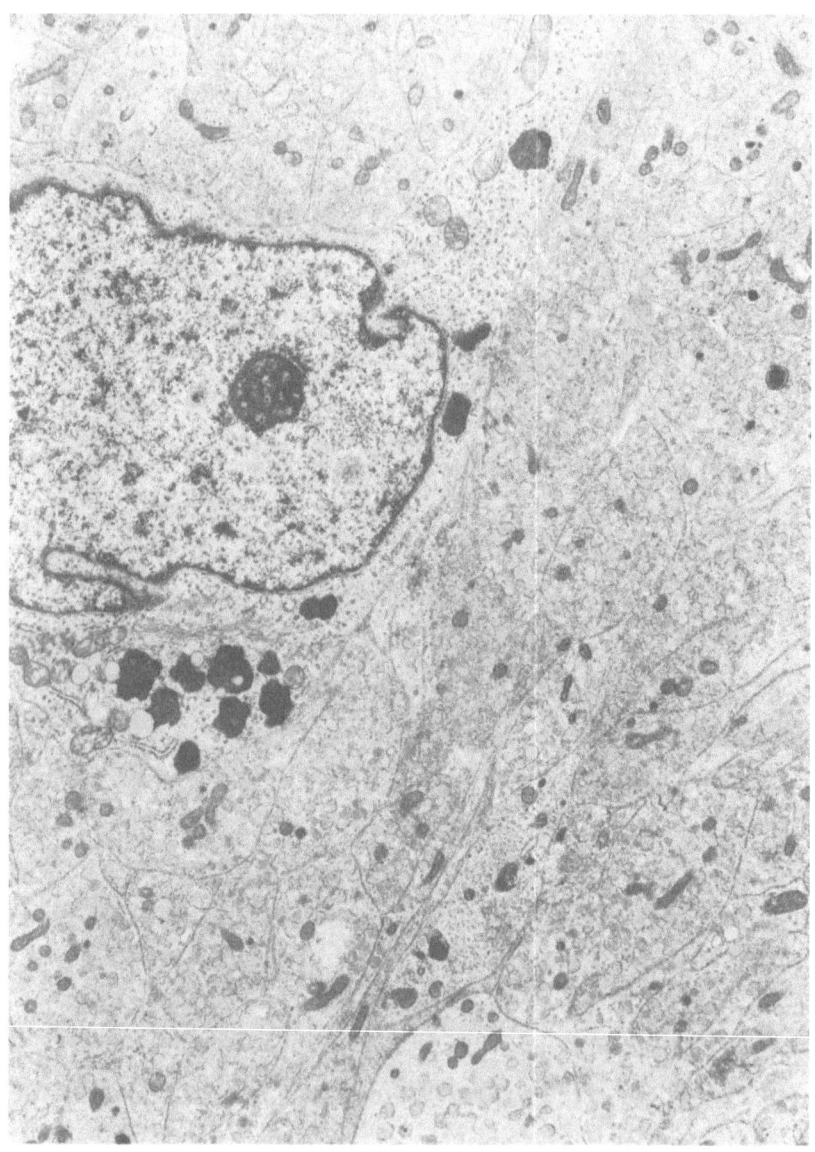

FIGURE 4. Electron micrograph of the posterior lobe showing a pituicyte. 8200 × .

2. PATHOLOGY

Clinically significant diseases of the posterior lobe are uncommon. From the endocrine standpoint, they can be divided into conditions caused by increased or decreased vasopressin secretion.

Inappropriate secretion of vasopressin, or Schwartz–Bartter syndrome, is characterized by renal sodium loss and hyponatremia and is due either to excessive vasopressin release from the posterior pituitary or to ectopic production by extrahypophysial neoplasms.[23–25] Ectopic vasopressin synthesis may be apparent in association with various malignant tumors, chiefly bronchogenic carcinoma. In some patients, no tumor is found, consistent with the view that vasopressin is discharged in excess from the posterior pituitary. Various diseases may be accompanied by increased vasopressin release, such as meningitis, myxedema, or cerebral lesions. The morphologic alterations within the hypothalamus, stalk, and posterior pituitary of patients with the nonneoplastic form of inappropriate vasopressin secretion have yet to be elucidated.

Diabetes insipidus is due to vasopressin deficiency and is characterized clinically by polyuria and polydipsia.[24,26] It may develop in patients with organic lesions of the hypothalamus, pituitary stalk, or posterior lobe that interfere with the synthesis of vasopressin, its transport from hypothalamic production sites to the posterior lobe, or its release from the posterior lobe. Morphologically, diverse lesions can be evident in the hypothalamus, especially within the nucleus supraopticus, the principal site of vasopressin synthesis, or along the supraopticohypophysial tract. Destruction of the posterior lobe results in only slight or moderate temporary polyuria and polydipsia. Organic lesions include various tumors, metastatic carcinomas, granulomas, traumatic injuries, histiocytosis X, meningoencephalitis, lymphomas, and leukemias. In the idiopathic form of diabetes insipidus, no gross destructive lesion can be demonstrated in the hypothalamus, stalk, or posterior lobe. Careful histologic study may reveal various organic abnormalities, such as reduction in size and number of the nerve cells of the supraoptic and paraventricular nuclei.[27]

The renal form of diabetes insipidus is attributed to end organ failure; the renal tubules are not capable of responding to the antidiuretic effect of vasopressin, leading to polyuria and polydipsia.[26] The disease is unassociated with hypothalamohypophysial lesions and vasopressin secretion is not impaired.

Aside from disturbance of water metabolism, abnormalities in the posterior pituitary, particularly space-occupying lesions, may cause local symptoms, such as headache and visual disturbances. The intracranial pressure may increase, producing anterior pituitary compression. Damage to the pituitary stalk may interrupt the portal circulation. The resultant arrest of adenohypophysial blood flow may lead to infarction in the anterior lobe and to changes in adenohypophysial endocrine activity.[28,29] Extensive loss of adenohypophysial tissue may result in various degrees of anterior hypopituitarism.[30]

The review of pathologic changes in the neurohypophysis will be based on their morphologic appearance.

Basophilic cell invasion is a common histologic finding in pituitaries obtained at unselected autopsies[7] (Figure 5). In the majority of cases, only a few basophilic cells are noted in the posterior lobe. In a few cases, however,

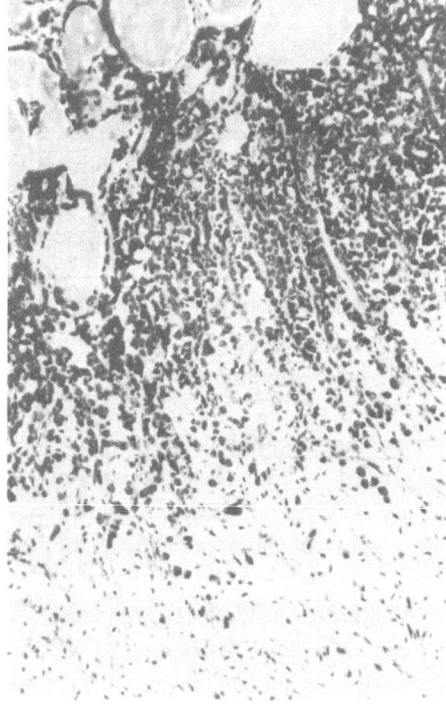

FIGURE 5. Basophilic cells spread deeply into the posterior lobe. Hematoxylin–phloxin–saffron. 100 × .

large groups of basophilic cells permeate the neural lobe.[31] The cytoplasm of such cells stains positively with basic dyes, exhibits varying degrees of periodic acid–Schiff (PAS) and lead–hematoxylin positivity, and yields strong staining for adrenocorticotropic hormone, β-LPH, and endorphins by the immunoperoxidase technique, indicating that they are corticotrophs. These cells differ from corticotrophs located in the anterior lobe; they are smaller and more dense than anterior lobe corticotrophs and, except for occasional cases, fail to show Crooke's hyalinization as a result of cortisol excess. Basophilic invasion does not occur before puberty and is more frequently seen in older subjects, especially aging men. It cannot be correlated with any endocrine abnormality and its significance is unknown. Even in cases with massive neurohypophysial corticotroph cell accumulation, no endocrine changes are manifest.

Squamous cell nests, glandular structures resembling salivary glands, and focal *lymphocytic infiltration* are common incidental findings in the posterior lobe or pituitary stalk.[32–34]

Hemorrhages and necroses are usually focal and uncommon.[35] They are associated with traumatic head injuries, postpartum necrosis of the anterior pituitary, increased intracranial pressure, shock, disseminated intravascular coagulation, septicemia, and various hematologic disorders. Clinical symptoms are rarely manifest, but diabetes insipidus may occur. Vessels in the neural lobe may contain hyaline thrombi in cases of thrombotic thrombocytopenic purpura (Figure 6).

Various *granulomas* (Figure 12) tuberculosis, sarcoidosis, and syphilis may be present in the stalk and the neural lobe.[36–39] Extensive tissue destruction may lead to diabetes insipidus.

The posterior lobe is frequently involved in histiocytosis X or Hand–Schüller–Christian disease[40–42] (Figure 13). Numerous eosinophilic leukocytes and lipid-laden foamy macrophages may be present or fibrosis may prevail. In some cases, the posterior lobe is completely destroyed and the pituitary stalk is also impaired. Diabetes insipidus is not infrequent in severe cases of histiocytosis X.[43]

Interruption of the pituitary stalk results in conspicuous morphologic changes along the entire supraopticohypophysial tract.[29,44] Surgical sectioning or traumatic disruption of the stalk results in atrophy of both the supraoptic and the paraventricular nuclei as well as of the posterior lobe. Various diseases can destroy the supraoptic and paraventricular nuclei or the supraopticohypophysial tract, thereby impairing the innervation of the posterior lobe. Since normal functional activity of the neurohypophysis depends upon the integrity

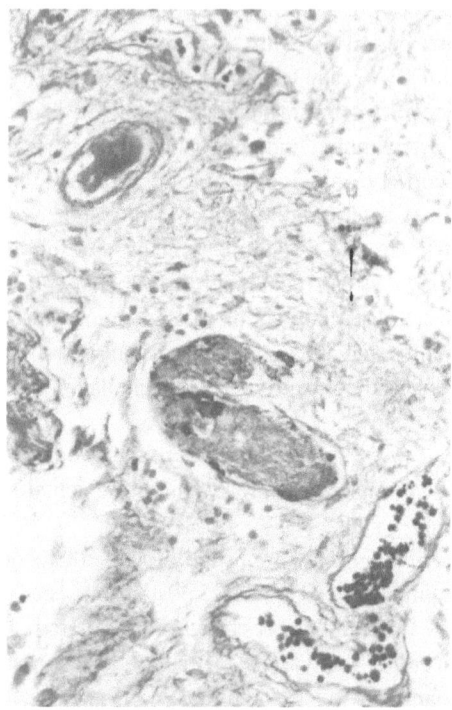

FIGURE 6. Thrombosis in the vessels of the posterior lobe in a case of thrombotic thrombo-cytopenic purpura. Phosphotungstic acid–hematoxylin. 250×.

of this nerve supply, interrupted innervation produces diabetes insipidus. Morphologically, the posterior lobe undergoes severe atrophy; the stainable neurosecretory material disappears, the tissue hormone content decreases to an unmeasurable amount, and the nervous tissue is replaced by a fibrous scar.

Involution of the neural lobe can also be seen in some cases of anterior hypopituitarism. In Sheehan's syndrome (postpartum hypopituitarism), neu-rohypophysial atrophy and involution of the supraoptic and paraventricular nuclei may be conspicuous.[45,46]

Neoplasms in the neurohypophysis are uncommon.

From the endocrinologic viewpoint, *secondary carcinomas* constitute the most important neoplasms[47-49] (Figures 7 and 15). Such metastases may represent incidental autopsy findings in cases of disseminated carcinomatosis. In these patients, tumor deposits can be detected in several organs, involve-ment of the neurohypophysis being clinically unrecognized. Nonetheless, in some patients with massive destruction of the neurohypophysis, diabetes insipidus develops, and polyuria as well as polydipsia is noted.[49-51]

Neurohypophysial metastases are not rare. The histologic study of pituitaries obtained at adult autopsies demonstrates secondary deposits in 1–3% of all cancer patients. The actual frequency of metastasis is probably higher, since small tumor deposits can easily be missed unless serial microsections are studied. A variety of neoplasms may give rise to metastases in the posterior pituitary, including carcinoma of the bronchus, breast, colon, and prostate; malignant melanoma; a variety of sarcomas; and hematopoietic malignancies including lymphoma, Hodgkin's disease, and leukemia[50] (Figure 14).

In comparison to their incidence in the adenohypophysis, carcinoma metastases occur more frequently in the neurohypophysis. This increased incidence is not unexpected in that, unlike the anterior lobe, the posterior pituitary has an extensive and direct arterial blood supply. Hence, metastases

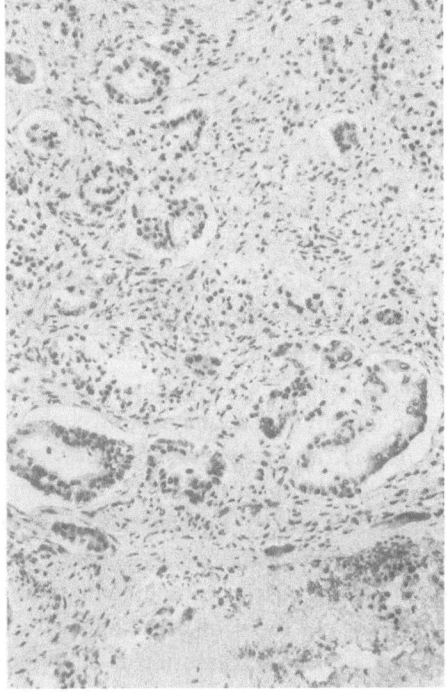

FIGURE 7. Metastatic adenocarcinoma in the posterior lobe. Hematoxylin–phloxin–saffron. 100×.

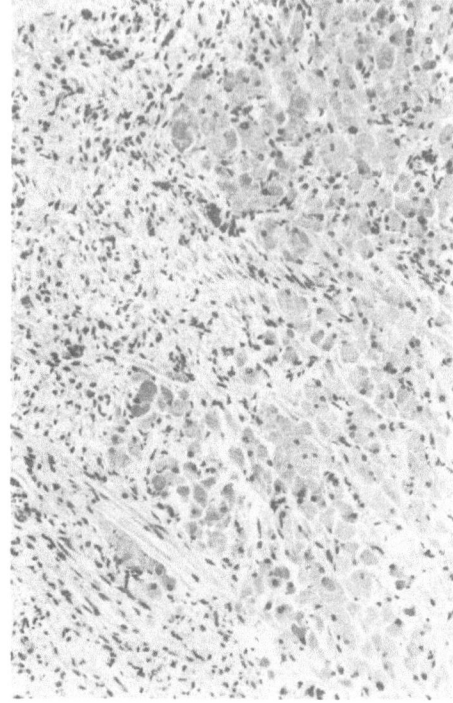

FIGURE 8. Granular cell tumor in the posterior lobe. Hematoxylin–phloxin–saffron. 100 ×.

can easily develop by a hematogenous route via the systemic circulation. In the majority of instances, metastases first occur in the neural lobe or pituitary stalk, the tumor spreading secondarily to the anterior lobe by direct extension or by the hematogenous route, via the portal vessels. Carcinomas from adjacent areas may also directly invade the neurohypophysis.

Granular cell tumors (also termed choristomas, granular cell myoblastomas, or tumorettes) are the most commonly occurring primary neurohypophysial tumors (Figures 8 and 9). Located most often in the posterior lobe and less commonly in the lower part of the hypophysial stalk, granular tumors have been noted in 1–8% of unselected adult autopsies, their incidence depending upon whether or not serial microsections are examined.[52] In most instances, such tumors are small, measuring 1–2 mm or even less, and are not evident on gross inspection. Granular cell tumors are slow growing, histologically benign, well demarcated but unencapsulated lesions, and are easily identified by light microscopy. The majority of granular cell tumors remain asymptomatic and are found incidentally at autopsy. Occasionally, however, they exhibit more rapid growth and may reach a large size, producing headache, visual disturbances, adenohypophysial insufficiency, and diabetes insipidus.[53,54] In exceptional cases, owing either to elevation of intracranial pressure or to cranial neuropathy, surgical removal of the tumor becomes necessary.[54,55]

Histologically, granular cell tumors are composed of loosely apposed large spherical, oval, or polygonal cells with eccentrically located nuclei and abundant acidophilic cytoplasm. Numerous large evenly distributed, strongly PAS-positive, luxol-fast-blue- and alcian-blue-positive granules almost fully occupy the cytoplasm and are a prominent feature.[56] The granules are rich in hydrolytic enzymes and have recently been shown to contain neuraminic acid as well as lectin receptors.[56] Immunoperoxidase stains have failed to

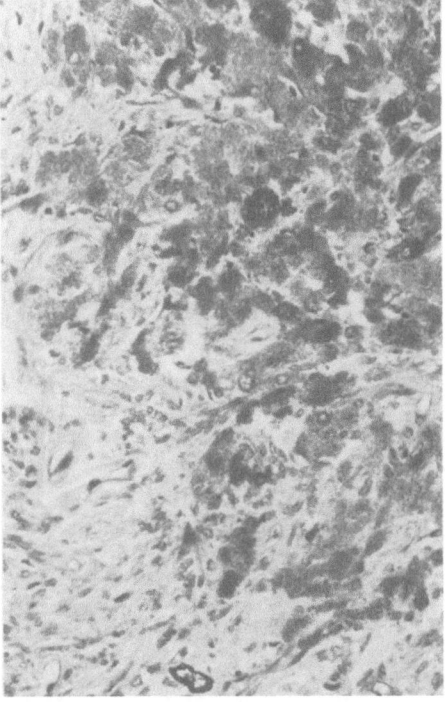

FIGURE 9. Cytoplasmic PAS-positive granules are apparent in a granular cell tumor of the posterior lobe. PAS technique. 250×.

demonstrate either adenohypophysial or neurohypophysial hormones. By electron microscopy, the granules are seen to represent large membrane-bound, unevenly electron-dense lysosomes.[57] Granular cell myoblastomas of other organs exhibit positive immunostaining for carcinoembryonic antigen.[58] It remains to be seen whether immunopositivity can be demonstrated in granular cell tumors of the posterior lobe.

The cytogenesis of granular cell tumors has yet to be established. In other organs, they are assumed to arise from Schwann cells or, less likely, from myoblasts. As far as the neurohypophysis is concerned, this theory is untenable, since these cell types do not occur in the normal posterior lobe. Choristomatous derivation would indicate misplacement of granular cells during the development of the pituitary. This hypothesis is, however, not supported by the fact that no neurohypophysial accumulation of granular cells occurs in younger subjects and that granular cell tumors can only be detected

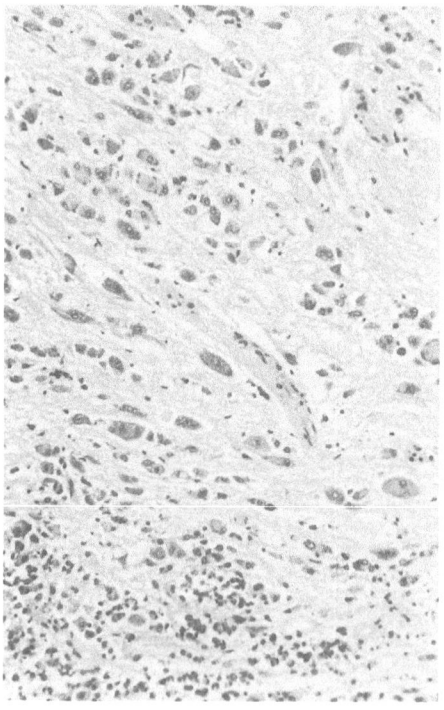

FIGURE 10. Infundibular hamartoma in association with a growth hormone cell adenoma of the pituitary, causing acromegaly. Hematoxylin–phloxin–saffron. 100 × .

in the posterior lobes of older men and women. The most obvious explanation is that granular cell tumors originate from pituicytes, the glial cells of the neural lobe.[59-61]

Beside granular cell tumors, *other neoplasms* originate very rarely in the neurohypophysis. Although on rare occasion gliomas may derive from the pituicytes and show an identical histologic appearance to glial tumors originating in the brain or spinal cord,[34,62] most gliomas affecting the neurohypophysis represent primarily lesions extending from the central nervous system. These tumors more commonly arise in the hypothalamus or median eminence and, by spreading downward, they invade the posterior lobe. In cases of massive destruction of the median eminence, pituitary stalk, or posterior lobe, diabetes insipidus may be apparent.

Few cases of gangliocytoma have been reported.[34] More work is required to establish correlations between morphologic features and clinical manifestations of this rare tumor type.

Neoplasms of the infundibulum are described under various names, such as infundibuloma, hamartoma, glioma, or astrocytoma.[63] These uncommon tumors, the majority being astrocytic in nature, are histologically benign and exhibit a slow growth rate. Occasionally, they may invade the pituitary stalk, neural lobe, or optic nerve and may extend to involve the mammillary bodies, hypothalamus, or third ventricle. By compression, displacement, or destruction of large portions of the hypothalamus, hypophysial stalk, or pituitary, such tumors may produce varied endocrinologic abnormalities, including various degrees of hypopituitarism, hyperprolactinemia, or diabetes insipidus. In some patients, obesity and hypogonadism may occur or precocious puberty may develop.[64,65]

Certain infundibular hamartomas may secrete luteinizing-hormone-releasing hormone (LHRH), and the resulting stimulation of adenohypophysial gonadotroph cells may cause increased discharge of gonadotroph hormones, accounting for premature sexual development. The presence of LHRH in the tumors can be demonstrated by immunocytologic techniques.[66] Occasionally, hypothalamic hamartomas are associated with pituitary growth hormone cell adenoma and acromegaly[67] (Figures 10 and 11). The secretion of growth-hormone-releasing substances responsible for growth hormone cell proliferation and increased growth hormone discharge is an intriguing possibility. Tumors arising in the pancreatic islets, bronchial epithelium, or intestines are known to produce factors with growth-hormone-releasing activity.[68-72] It remains to be determined whether or not certain hypothalamic hamartomas possess similar abilities.

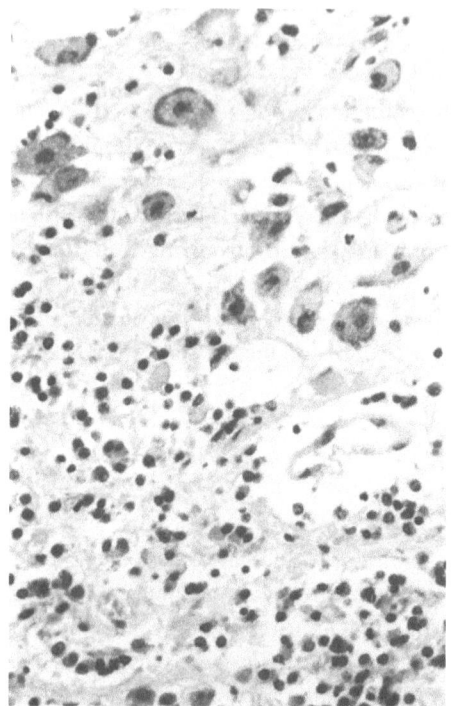

FIGURE 11. The same lesion as in Figure 10, showing nerve cells and adenomatous growth hormone cells. Hematoxylin–phloxin–saffron. 250 × .

3. SUMMARY

The salient features of neurohypophysial pathology have been summarized in this chapter. Although the posterior lobe is rarely the site of primary disease, several lesions may impair neurohypophysial structure and hormonal activity. From the endocrine point of view, diabetes insipidus is the most important abnormality. This rare syndrome is due to vasopressin deficiency and is characterized by polyuria and polydipsia. It may be associated with several anatomically different lesions that interfere with the functional integrity of certain areas of the hypothalamus, hypophysial stalk, or neural lobe.

ACKNOWLEDGMENTS. This work was supported in part by Grant MA-6349 from the Medical Research Council of Canada. The author wishes to thank Mrs. Wanda Wlodarski for excellent secretarial work.

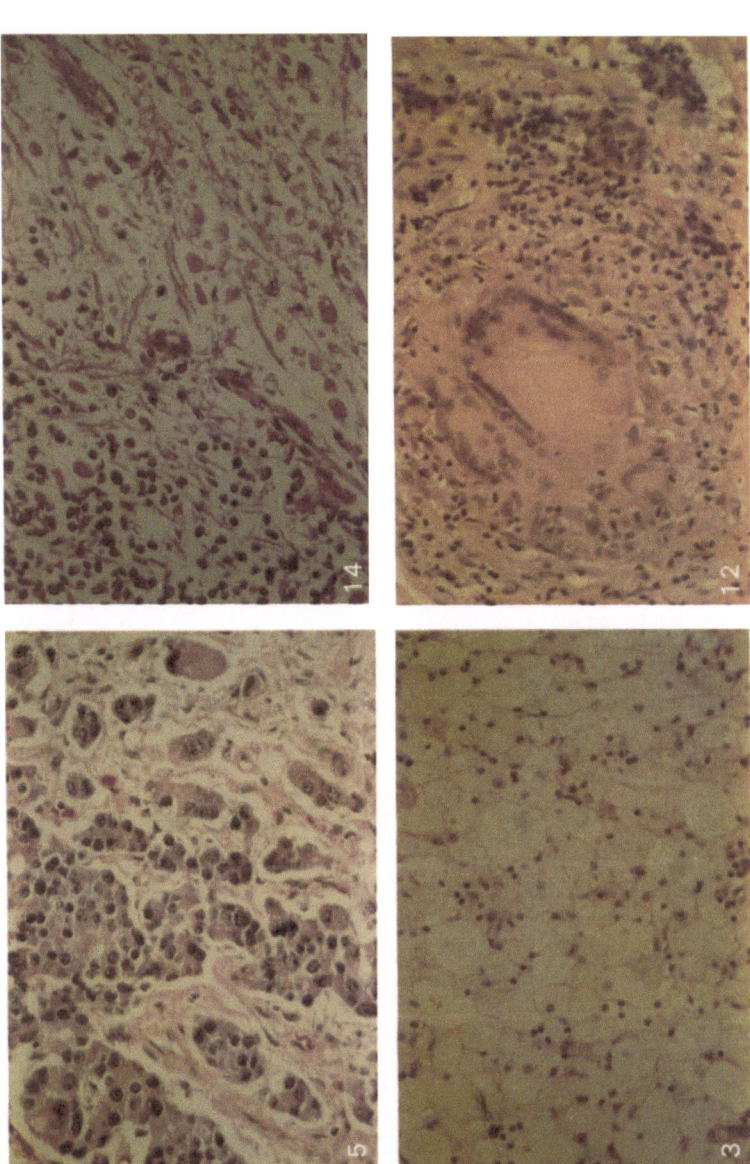

FIGURE 12. Giant-cell granuloma replacing the pituitary gland. Hematoxylin–eosin. 250 ×, reproduced at 225%.

FIGURE 13. Histiocytosis X destroying large areas of the posterior lobe of the pituitary as well as the hypophysial stalk and causing diabetes insipidus. Hematoxylin–phloxin–saffron. 250 ×, reproduced at 225%.

FIGURE 14. Malignant lymphoma in the posterior lobe of the pituitary. Hematoxylin–phloxin–saffron. 250 ×, reproduced at 225%.

FIGURE 15. Metastatic carcinoma in the posterior lobe of the pituitary. Hematoxylin–phloxin–saffron. 250 ×, reproduced at 225%.

REFERENCES

1. Watkins WB: Localization of neurosecretory pathways in the hypothalamus. *Prog Neuropathol* 3:383, 1976.
2. Sandow J: Location of hypothalamic control centres and nature of regulatory hormones. *Clin Endocrinol Metab* 6:155, 1977.
3. Zimmerman EA: Localization of hormone secreting pathways in the brain by immunohistochemistry and light microscopy: A review. *Fed Proc* 36:1964, 1977.
4. Brownstein MJ, Russell JT, Gainer H: Synthesis, transport and release of posterior pituitary hormones. *Science* 207:373, 1980.
5. Alonso G, Gabrion J, Travers E, et al: Ultrastructural organization of actin filaments in neurosecretory axons of the rat. *Cell Tissue Res* 214:323, 1981.
6. Decherney A, Naftolin F: Hypothalamic and pituitary development in the fetus. *Clin Obstet Gynecol* 23:749, 1980.
7. Horvath E, Kovacs K: Pathology of the pituitary gland, in Ezrin C, Horvath E, Kaufman B (eds): *Pituitary Diseases*. Boca Raton, Florida, CRC Press, 1980, pp 1–83.
8. Okado N, Yokota N: An electron microscopic study on the structural development of the neural lobe in the human fetus. *Am J Anat* 159:261, 1980.
9. Silverman AJ: Ultrastructural studies on the localization of neurohypophysial hormones and their carrier proteins. *J Histochem Cytochem* 24:816, 1976.
10. Dierickx K, Vandesande F: Immunocytochemical localization of the vasopressinergic and the oxytocinergic neurons in the human hypothalamus. *Cell Tissue Res* 184:15, 1977.
11. Dierickx K, Vandesande F: Immunocytochemical demonstration of separate vasopressin-neurophysin and oxytocin-neurophysin neurons in the human hypothalamus. *Cell Tissue Res* 196:203, 1979.
12. Dierickx K: Immunocytochemical localization of the vertebrate cyclic nonapeptide neurohypophyseal hormones and neurophysins. *Int Rev Cytol* 62:119, 1980.
13. Vandesande F, Dierickx K, Goossens N: Immunocytochemical localization of the posterior lobe hormones and of their carrier proteins. *J Histochem Cytochem* 28:469, 1980.
14. Bergland RM, Torack RM: An electron microscopic study of the human infundibulum. *Z Zellforsch* 99:1, 1969.
15. Kobayashi H, Matsui T, Ishii S: Functional electron microscopy of the hypothalamic median eminence. *Int Rev Cytol* 29:281, 1970.
16. Dellmann HD: Degeneration and regeneration of neurosecretory systems. *Int Rev Cytol* 36:215, 1973.
17. Bloodworth JMB Jr, Horvath E, Kovacs K: Fine structural pathology of the endocrine system, in Trump BF, Jones RT (eds): *Diagnostic Electron Microscopy*. New York, John Wiley and Sons, 1980, vol 3, pp 359–527.
18. Seyama S, Pearl GS, Takei Y: Ultrastructural study of the human neurohypophysis. I. Neurosecretory axons and their dilatations in the pars nervosa. *Cell Tissue Res* 205:253, 1980.
19. Seyama S, Pearl GS, Takei Y: Ultrastructural study of the human neurohypophysis. III. Vascular and perivascular structures. *Cell Tissue Res* 206:291, 1980.
20. Takei Y, Seyama S, Pearl GS, et al: Ultrastructural study of the human neurohypophysis. II. Cellular elements of neural parenchyma, the pituicytes. *Cell Tissue Res* 205:273, 1980.
21. Bergland RM, Page RB: Pituitary–brain vascular relations: A new paradigm. *Science* 204:18, 1979.
22. Krieger DT, Liotta AS: Pituitary hormones in brain: Where, how, and why? *Science* 205:366, 1979.

23. De Troyer A, Demanet JC: Clinical, biological and pathogenic features of the syndrome of inappropriate secretion of antidiuretic hormone. A review of 26 cases with marked hyponatraemia. *Q J Med* 45:521, 1976.
24. Krieger DT: Central nervous system disease. *Clin Endocrinol Metab* 8:467, 1979.
25. Lester MC, Nelson PB: Neurological aspects of vasopressin release and the syndrome of inappropriate secretion of antidiuretic hormone. *Neurosurgery* 8:735, 1981.
26. Kleeman CR, Berl T: The neurohypophysial hormones: Vasopressin, in DeGroot LJ, Cahill GF Jr, Martini L (eds): *Endocrinology*. New York, Grune and Stratton, 1979, vol 1, pp 253–275.
27. Green JR, Buchan GC, Alvord EC Jr, et al: Hereditary and idiopathic types of diabetes insipidus. *Brain* 90:707, 1967.
28. Adams JH, Daniel PM, Prichard MML: Transection of the pituitary stalk in man: Anatomical changes in the pituitary glands of 21 patients. *J Neurol Neurosurg Psychiat* 29:545, 1966.
29. Daniel PM, Prichard MML: Studies of the hypothalamus and the pituitary gland with special reference to the effects of transection of the pituitary stalk. *Acta Endocrinol* 80 (Suppl. 201):1, 1975.
30. Kovacs K: Necrosis of anterior pituitary in humans. *Neuroendocrinology* 4:170, 201, 1969.
31. Rasmussen AT: Origin of the basophilic cells in the posterior lobe of the human hypophysis. *Am J Anat* 46:461, 1930.
32. Schochet SS Jr, McCormick WF, Halmi NS: Salivary gland nests in the human pituitary. Light and electron microscopical study. *Arch Pathol* 98:193, 1974.
33. Asa SL, Kovacs K, Bilbao JM, et al: Immunohistochemical localization of keratin in craniopharyngiomas and squamous cell nests of the human pituitary. *Acta Neuropathol* 54:257, 1981.
34. Sheehan HL, Kovacs K: Neurohypophysis and hypothalamus, in Bloodworth JMB Jr (ed): *Endocrine Pathology*. Baltimore, Williams and Wilkins, 1982, pp 45–99.
35. Kornblum RN, Fisher RS: Pituitary lesions in craniocerebral injuries. *Arch Pathol* 88:242, 1969.
36. Brust JCM, Rhee RS, Plank CR, et al: Sarcoidosis, galactorrhea, and amenorrhea: 2 autopsy cases, 1 with Chiari–Frommel syndrome. *Ann Neurol* 2:130, 1977.
37. Delaney P: Neurologic manifestations in sarcoidosis. Review of the literature, with a report of 23 cases. *Ann Intern Med* 87:336, 1977.
38. Stuart CA, Neelon FA, Lebovitz HE: Hypothalamic insufficiency: The cause of hypopituitarism in sarcoidosis. *Ann Intern Med* 88:589, 1978.
39. Del Pozo JM, Roda JE, Montoya JG, et al: Intrasellar granuloma. Case report. *J Neurosurg* 53:717, 1980.
40. Ezrin C, Chaikoff R, Hoffman H: Panhypopituitarism caused by Hand–Schüller–Christian disease. *Can Med Assoc J* 89:1290, 1963.
41. Helbock H, Krivit W, Nesbit ME Jr: Patterns of antidiuretic function in diabetes insipidus caused by histiocytosis-X. *J Lab Clin Med* 78:194, 1971.
42. Goodman RH, Post KD, Molitch ME, et al: Eosinophilic granuloma mimicking a pituitary tumor. *Neurosurgery* 5:723, 1979.
43. Daniel PM, Treip CS: The pathology of the hypothalamus. *Clin Endocrinol Metab* 6:3, 1977.
44. Daniel PM, Prichard MML: The human hypothalamus and pituitary stalk after hypophysectomy or pituitary stalk section. *Brain* 95:813, 1972.
45. Sheehan HL, Whitehead R: The neurohypophysis in post-partum hypopituitarism. *J Pathol Bact* 85:145, 1963.
46. Whitehead R: The hypothalamus in post-partum hypopituitarism. *J Pathol Bact* 86:55, 1963.
47. Duchen LW: Metastatic carcinoma in the pituitary gland and hypothalamus. *J Pathol Bact* 91:347, 1966.

48. Kovacs K: Metastatic cancer of the pituitary gland. *Oncology* 27:533, 1973.
49. Houck WA, Olson KB, Horton J: Clinical features of tumor metastasis to the pituitary. *Cancer* 26:656, 1970.
50. Teears RJ, Silverman EM: Clinicopathologic review of 88 cases of carcinoma metastatic to the pituitary gland. *Cancer* 36:216, 1975.
51. Yap HY, Tashima CK, Glumenschein GR, et al: Diabetes insipidus and breast cancer. *Arch Intern Med* 139:1009, 1979.
52. Luse SA, Kernohan JW: Granular cell tumors of the stalk and posterior lobe of the pituitary gland. *Cancer* 8:616, 1955.
53. Schlachter LB, Tindall GT, Pearl GS: Granular cell tumor of the pituitary gland associated with diabetes insipidus. *Neurosurgery* 6:418, 1980.
54. Becker DH, Wilson CB: Symptomatic parasellar granular cell tumors. *Neurosurgery* 8:173, 1981.
55. Satyamurti S, Huntington HW: Granular cell myoblastoma of the pituitary. Case report. *J Neurosurg* 37:483, 1972.
56. Muller W, Klein PJ, Newman RA, et al: Histochemical methods for the further characterization of the tumourettes of the posterior lobe of the pituitary. *Acta Neuropathol* 49:101, 1980.
57. Popovitch ER, Sutton CH, Besker NH, et al: Fine structure and histochemical studies of choristomas of the neurohypophysis. *J Neuropathol Exp Neurol* 29:155, 1970.
58. Shousha S, Lyssiotis T: Granular cell myoblastoma: Positive staining for carcinoembryonic antigen. *J Clin Pathol* 32:219, 1979.
59. Burston J, John R, Spencer H: "Myoblastoma" of the neurohypophysis. *J Pathol Bact* 83:455, 1962.
60. Jenevein EP: A neurohypophyseal tumor originating from pituicytes. *Am J Clin Pathol* 41:522, 1964.
61. Massie AP: A granular-cell pituicytoma of the neurohypophysis. *J Pathol* 129:53, 1979.
62. Scothorne CM: A glioma of the posterior lobe of the pituitary gland. *J Pathol Bact* 69:109, 1955.
63. Wolman L: Infundibuloma. *J Pathol Bact* 77:283, 1959.
64. Wolman L, Balmforth GV: Precocious puberty due to a hypothalamic hamartoma in a patient surviving to late middle age. *J Neurol Neurosurg Psychiat* 26:275, 1963.
65. Northfield DWC, Russell DS: Pubertas praecox due to hypothalamic hamartoma: Report of two cases surviving surgical removal of the tumour. *J Neurol Neurosurg Psychiat* 30:166, 1967.
66. Judge DM, Kulin HE, Page R, et al: Hypothalamic hamartoma. A source of luteinizing-hormone-releasing factor in precocious puberty. *N Engl J Med* 296:7, 1977.
67. Asa S, Bilbao JM, Kovacs K, et al: Hypothalamic neuronal hamartoma associated with pituitary growth hormone cell adenoma and acromegaly. *Acta Neuropathol* 52:231, 1980.
68. Caplan RH, Koob L, Abellera RM, et al: Cure of acromegaly by operative removal of an islet cell tumor of the pancreas. *Am J Med* 64:874, 1978.
69. Saeed uz Zafar M, Mellinger RC, Fine G, et al: Acromegaly associated with a bronchial carcinoid tumor: Evidence for ectopic production of growth hormone-releasing activity. *J Clin Endocrinol Metab* 48:66, 1979.
70. Shalet SM, Beardwell CG, MacFarlane IA, et al: Acromegaly due to production of a growth hormone releasing factor by a bronchial carcinoid tumour. *Clin Endocrinol* 10:61, 1979.
71. Frohman LA, Szabo M, Berelowitz M, et al: Partial purification and characterization of a peptide with growth hormone-releasing activity from extrapituitary tumors in patients with acromegaly. *J Clin Invest* 65:43, 1980.
72. Leveston SA, McKeel DW Jr, Buckley PJ, et al: Acromegaly and Cushing's syndrome associated with a foregut carcinoid tumor. *J Clin Endocrinol Metab* 53:682, 1981.

7

CLINICAL AND LABORATORY FEATURES OF CENTRAL AND NEPHROGENIC DIABETES INSIPIDUS AND PRIMARY POLYDIPSIA

Arnold M. Moses

1. CLINICAL FEATURES

In the last nine years, using modern techniques, I have investigated over 100 patients with long-standing central diabetes insipidus, defined as being present more than 6 months or until the patient died (Table I). The median age of onset was 22.5 years and 60% of the patients were male. The largest group was idiopathic (27%), followed closely by patients who developed diabetes insipidus before or after surgery for primary brain (extrapituitary) tumors (26%). Patients who developed diabetes insipidus following head trauma constituted the third largest group (18%). Eight percent of the patients had metastatic tumors of the hypothalamus, and 7% of the patients developed diabetes insipidus following hypophysectomy for treatment of pituitary hypersecretion, diabetic retinopathy, or cancer. Five percent developed diabetes insipidus before or after surgery for nonfunctioning pituitary tumors and the same number developed the disease from cerebral hypoperfusion. Four percent had histocytosis and the remaining cases were due to sarcoidosis or to a ruptured cerebral aneurysm. Rare causes which have been reported but which

Arnold M. Moses • Veterans Administration Medical Center and Department of Medicine, State University of New York, Upstate Medical Center, Syracuse, New York 13210.

TABLE I. 104 Cases of Long-standing Central Diabetes Insipidus Diagnosed in the Past 9 yr at SUNY, Upstate Medical Center[a]

Cause	Number of cases	Males	Females	Median age of onset	Range (yr)
Histiocytosis	4	2	2	2	1–20
Primary brain tumor[b]					
Postoperative DI	13	6	7	12	2–25
Preoperative DI	14	12	2	17	3–58
Idiopathic	28	19	9	17	Infancy to 66
Head trauma	18	12	6	22	5–48
Anoxemic encephalopathy	5	2	3	37	15–73
Nonfunctioning pituitary tumor (pre- or postoperative)	5	4	1	38	15–41
Ruptured cerebral aneurysm	1	1	0	39	
Sarcoidosis	1	0	1	42	
Posthypophysectomy for treatment of Cushing's syndrome, acromegaly, diabetic retinopathy, cancer	7	1	6	46	24–68
Metastatic malignancy	8	5	3	57	32–71

[a] Categories arranged in order of increasing median age of onset.
[b] Group consisted of 16 patients with craniopharyngeomas, 6 with pinealomas, and 5 with gliomas.

we have not observed include thrombotic thrombocytopenic purpura,[1] pituitary apoplexy,[2] Wegener's granulomatosis,[3] and systemic blastomycosis.[4]

One third of the patients who were classified in Table I as having idiopathic diabetes insipidus had one or more additional abnormalities (Table II). The other endocrine abnormalities probably reflect hypothalamic disease beyond the supraoptic and/or paraventricular nuclei. A thickened infundibular stalk on CT scan of the brain has previously been reported in patients with diabetes insipidus,[5] but there is no information available pertaining to the relationship of this finding to the cause of the diabetes insipidus. It is my belief that in the future patients with diabetes insipidus with any of the findings listed in Table II should be classified as having diabetes insipidus, cause to

be determined. These patients should be examined more frequently and carefully than patients who have no abnormalities other than diabetes insipidus.

Idiopathic diabetes insipidus usually occurs sporadically but may be
inherited either as an autosomal dominant or as an X-linked recessive disorder.[6] In five members of a single family with hereditary diabetes insipidus,
arginine vasopressin (AVP) and its specific neurophysin have been shown to
be absent from the urine and serum respectively, while oxytocin and its
neurophysin were sometimes present.[7] Pathology studies in several patients
with idiopathic diabetes insipidus, including the inherited type, have disclosed
a striking depletion of the Nissl granules and of the number of neurons in the
supraoptic and paraventricular nuclei.[6]

Idiopathic diabetes insipidus is almost always permanent. However, we
did have one patient with idiopathic diabetes insipidus who spontaneously
reverted to normal after approximately 10 months of the disease.

Diabetes insipidus is a well recognized complication of blunt head trauma.
The clinical data on 18 of our patients who had this problem for more than
6 months or until they died are listed on Table III. This type of diabetes
insipidus is occurring with increasing frequency, probably because of improved medical care for head trauma victims, which has resulted in survival
of patients who previously would have died from severe neurological damage.
The problem is usually recognized as early as 12–24 hr following the accident.[8] Delays in diagnosis occur when head trauma does not appear to be
severe, when the patient is admitted to a surgical service other than neurosurgery, or when the patient has unrecognized adrenal insufficiency. Since

TABLE II. Additional Endocrinological,
Neurological, or Radiological Findings
in Nine of the Patients Classified as
Having Idiopathic Diabetes Insipidus

4	Thyroid-stimulating hormone deficiency
3	Galactorrhea or increased prolactin levels
2	Growth hormone deficiency
2	ACTH deficiency
2	Gonadotropin deficiency
2	Thickened infundibular stalk on CT scan
1	Questionably enlarged sella turcica
1	Abnormal cerebrospinal fluid
1	Narcolepsy
1	Cerebral palsy

TABLE III. Clinical Data on 18 Patients with Long-standing Traumatic Diabetes Insipidus

Age of onset: Median 22 yr; range 5–48 yr

Sex: 12 M, 6 F

Cause

   Automobile accident: 13

   Fall from bicycle, motorcycle accident, industrial explosion, falling house, falling tree: 1 each

Skull fracture: 13

Permanent[a] endocrine abnormality (other than DI):   8

   Deficient thyroid-stimulating hormone: 5

   Deficient gonadotropins: 5

   Deficient ACTH: 3

   Deficient human growth hormone: 3

   Increased prolactin: 4

Permanent[a] neurological damage: 9

   Cranial nerves: 8

      First cranial nerve: 3

      Second cranial nerve or optic chiasm: 6

      Other cranial nerves: 3

   Hemiparesis: 2

   Massive diffuse brain damage, carotid–cavernous fistula, adipisia, ataxia: 1 each

Loss of consciousness: None in 1 patient, minutes to months in remainder

[a] Greater than 6 months.

glucocorticoids are essential for the development of marked hypotonic poly-uria,[9-13] the diabetes insipidus in these patients becomes evident only after the initiation of steroid therapy. A question may arise about trauma as a possible cause of diabetes insipidus when multiple head injuries occur in someone like a professional boxer, especially if symptoms are first noted weeks or months after his last fight. The diabetes insipidus caused by trauma may persist for anywhere from several hours to the duration of the patient's life. It is generally considered that traumatic diabetes insipidus will be per-manent if the patient does not recover by 4–6 months. However, we have had patients who improved to the point of not requiring therapy after intervals of 2 years, 3 years, and 10 years. I will describe in more detail one of our cases who continued to improve for at least $2^1/_2$ years (Figure 1). During that period his urine concentration improved in relation to his plasma osmolality, his urine volume decreased from 11.1 to 1.76 liters/days and his saline-induced osmotic threshold (see Section 2) decreased from 314.8 to 291.3 mOsm/kg. Therapy was discontinued between the second and third dehydration tests. The patient's serum sodium concentration remained slightly elevated. When patients like this have partial antidiuretic hormone (ADH) deficiency, as he did between the second and third dehydration tests, the sensitivity of the thirst

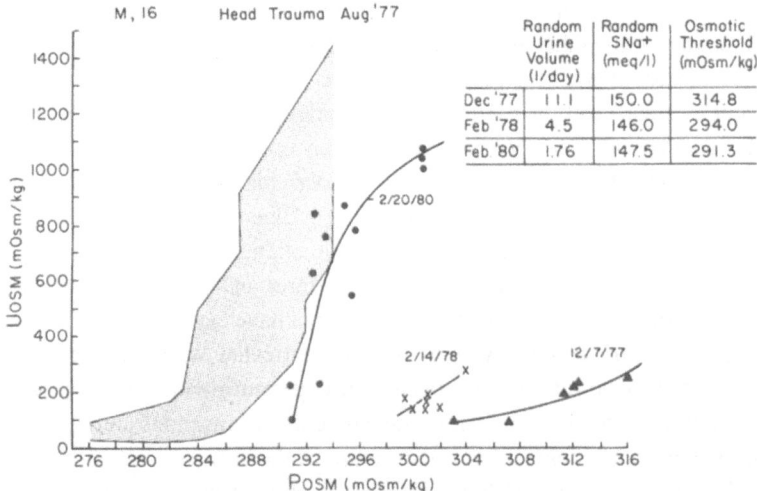

FIGURE 1. Changes in plasma versus urine osmolality coordinates over a 26-month period in a patient with traumatic diabetes insipidus. Note that the improvement in urine concentration in relation to plasma osmolality was associated with a marked decrease in urine volume and osmotic threshold and with an associated decrease but not normalization of the serum sodium concen-tration.

mechanism determines the degree of polydipsia and polyuria. Since patients like this can concentrate urine with a supranormal osmotic stimulus, they may have severe polydipsia and polyuria if the thirst mechanism is sensitive, or a high-set osmoreceptor or essential hypernatremia if the thirst sensation is blunted. The problem of hypernatremia in patients or animal models with defective AVP release has been discussed in detail.[9]

Most of our patients who developed long-standing traumatic diabetes insipidus had substantial neurological damage (Table III). There was a high incidence of damage to the first and second cranial nerves. Three of our patients had loss of smell, while six had damage to the optic nerves or chiasm. Savino et al. reported that half of their patients who were evaluated for traumatic chiasmal syndromes developed diabetes insipidus at least transiently.[14] A total of nine of our patients had permanent neurological damage, while 13 had one or more skull fractures. There are cases, however, in whom the diabetes insipidus developed shortly after very minimal trauma. The amount of trauma to our patients has ranged from a fall from a bicycle, causing only transitory unconsciousness and no skull fracture, to unconsciousness for longer than 5 months associated with low EEG activity. Thus, although substantial head trauma may alert the physician to anticipate diabetes insipidus as a complication, it may occur with any head injury.

Detailed assessment of anterior pituitary function in patients with traumatic diabetes insipidus usually requires a delay until the patient is medically stable. Almost all of these patients initially receive adrenal steroid therapy to prevent or treat cerebral edema, and the detailed evaluation of thyroid, gonadal, and growth hormone function is often impractical or difficult during the initial hospitalization period. The endocrinological data that could be obtained in our patients with long-standing traumatic diabetes insipidus are listed in Table III. We should remember that adrenal insufficiency masks the manifestations of ADH deficiency, and the three patients with adrenocorticotropic hormone (ACTH) deficiency would not have expressed the hypotonic polyuria of ADH deficiency until they were treated with glucocorticoids. Barreca et al. have recently reviewed their experience with anterior pituitary abnormalities in ten patients with traumatic diabetes insipidus and found that eight patients were deficient in one or more of the anterior lobe hormones.[15]

Anoxemia or cerebral hypoperfusion is another cause of diabetes insipidus that is being described more frequently. At least nine cases have been reported in the past,[16-20] and we have studied five additional patients (Table IV). The previously reported patients had severe encephalomalacia almost

TABLE IV. Clinical Data on Five Patients Who Developed Diabetes Insipidus from Anoxemic Encephalopathy[a]

Patient data	Cause	Time of development of diabetes insipidus
M, 15	Gunshot wound of chest causing shock	24–36 hr after injury, which caused marked neurological abnormalities, including bilateral fixed dilated pupils and absence of respiration
F, 32	Embolus to left middle cerebral artery and uncal herniation	$2^1/_2$ days after initial paresis; about 12 hr after fixed, dilated pupils and decerebrate posturing
F, 37	Hypertensive encephalopathy	2 days after hyperreflexia and muscle twitching, 1 day after occipital blindness and severe obtundation, and 2–3 hr after development of severe brain stem dysfunction
M, 49[b]	Cardiopulmonary arrest	About 3 hr after the arrest and development of brain death
F, 73	Cardiopulmonary arrest	24 hr after the arrest, which caused fixed, dilated pupils, absent reflexes and respiration, and failure of oculovestibular responses

[a] All patients had to be maintained on total life support systems and were brain dead at the time diabetes insipidus developed.
[b] Developed panhypopituitarism. Remainder of patients could not be evaluated for anterior pituitary function.

always associated with brain death resulting from asphyxia, drug-induced respiratory failure, diabetic ketoacidosis, cardiac arrest, or shock due to penetrating thoracic trauma. Our five patients (two males, three females) ranged in age from 15 to 73 years and developed encephalopathy and diabetes insipidus from shock secondary to a gunshot wound of the chest, an embolus to the middle cerebral artery, hypertensive encephalopathy, and cardiopulmonary arrest. One of our patients, who survived for 68 days after the criteria for brain death were satisfied, had findings at autopsy that were characteristic of an advanced stage in the sequence of changes that follow brain infarction with prolonged preservation of systemic circulatory function.[21]

Only one of our patients had sarcoidosis. However, diabetes insipidus has been reported by others in patients with sarcoidosis.[22,23] Sarcoidosis may also cause primary polydipsia and acquired nephrogenic diabetic insipidus.[24,25]

Diabetic insipidus resulted from metastatic malignancy in eight cases. There were two cases each with carcinoma of lung and breast, and one case each from carcinoma of kidney and rectum, one carcinoma with an unknown primary site, and one patient with leukemia. Diabetes insipidus as a complication of leukemia, though rare, has been previously reported.[26,27] Thirty-nine cases of metastatic breast carcinoma causing diabetic insipidus have been reported by Yap et al.[28]

Hypernatremia may develop with either a concentrated or a dilute urine. There may be an intact neurohypophysial system with an unavailability of water, or there may be vasopressin deficiency of varying degrees for several reasons. Some patients may have a defective osmoreceptor mechanism while volume receptor mechanisms remain intact.[29-32] The osmotic threshold for vasopressin release may be absent or elevated.[33] For hypernatremia to develop, thirst perception must be defective or water must be unavailable to the patient.[34] The majority of patients with myotonic dystrophy may have asymptomatic hypernatremia due to ineffective osmoreceptor function with intact volume control of AVP release in association with a deficient thirst mechanism.[35] We have found a similar situation in two patients with Kallmann's syndrome.

We have had five patients with inability to concentrate urine even with very high levels of serum sodium who had no sense of thirst (Table V). The clinical problem presented by these patients is severe. It is very impressive and frightening to have one of these patients obtunded or in shock with a serum sodium of 180 mEq/liter and absolutely no sensation of thirst. The patients can be maintained in the hospital with some difficulty by careful adjustment of fluid intake on the basis of urine volume and estimated insensible and sensible fluid losses, with modifications made according to body weight and serum electrolyte and osmolality determinations. However, it is very

TABLE V. Clinical Features of Conscious Patients with Diabetes Insipidus and Hypodipsia

Patient data	Cause	Duration of hypodipsia
M, 12	Following surgery for pinealoma	Permanent
M, 16	Head trauma	2–3 months
M, 18	Pinealoma	Permanent
M, 22	Head trauma	Permanent
M, 39	Ruptured cerebral aneurysm	Permanent

difficult to do this at home and the results may be very poor unless there is a nurse in constant attendance or the lay person caring for the patient is highly motivated and has good insight. Although Bode et al. reported that chlorpropamide may restore drinking behavior,[36] it has not been successful in our patients.

Nephrogenic diabetes insipidus is a form of hypotonic polyuria that is usually characterized by almost total resistance to the antidiuretic action of vasopressin. We have, however, investigated a 29-year-old female who concentrated her urine to greater than 400 mOsm/kg following the subcutaneous injection of 8 μg of 1-desamine-8-D-arginine vasopressin (dDAVP). Patients like this can be very difficult to distinguish from those with central diabetes insipidus unless AVP levels are measured. In patients with nephrogenic diabetes insipidus the hormonal resistance and subsequent dehydration result in high plasma and urine levels of AVP. The inability to concentrate urine may be due to failure either to form cyclic AMP (cAMP) in the kidney in response to ADH[37] or to concentrate urine in response to endogenously released cAMP, since there is no antidiuretic response to infused cAMP or dibutyryl cAMP.[38,39] There are major problems in investigating the renal abnormality in nephrogenic diabetes insipidus in man. Urinary cAMP in normal subjects increases only minimally even after large pressor doses of AVP, so that an impaired response is very difficult to detect, and the infusion of cAMP or dibutryl cAMP causes a variety of vascular and other metabolic changes that interfere with interpretation of the response.

Personal observations on two patients indicate that AVP normally increases systemic vascular resistance and urinary prostaglandin E excretion in patients with nephrogenic diabetes insipidus. ACTH is also released normally by ADH in these patients.[40] In contrast to one report,[37] we have not found renal resistance to the action of parathyroid hormone in these patients. It appears, therefore, that the defect in patients with nephrogenic diabetes insipidus who have been investigated is limited to failure of the antidiuretic response to ADH. Since vascular, ACTH-releasing, and renal-prostaglandin-stimulating actions of ADH are intact, the biochemical basis of this disease may be confined to an abnormality of the antidiuretic receptor of the medullary collecting tubule. A clear understanding of the precise abnormality in man will have to await studies of AVP binding, enzyme kinetics, and cyclic nucleotide metabolism in diseased kidneys.

Because of the difficulty in studying the biochemical basis of hereditary nephrogenic diabetes insipidus in man, several species of mice with this abnormality have been investigated. Valtin has reviewed this subject in detail.[41] In one species of mice Dousa and Valtin have found an impaired stimulation of renal medullary adenylate cyclase by vasopressin without an abnormality of cAMP-dependent protein kinase or content of microtubular subunits.[42] Subsequent experiments in this species have revealed that their unresponsiveness to vasopressin mainly results from the inability of collecting tubules to increase intracellular cAMP levels in response to vasopressin. This, in turn, may be at least partly the result of an abnormally high phosphodiesterase activity combined with a lower activity of vasopressin-sensitive adenylate cyclase activity.[43]

Hereditary nephrogenic diabetes insipidus in man is a rare disorder, usually manifested in males, but with X-linked transmission. Many North American patients with this disorder can trace their ancestry to settlers who arrived in Nova Scotia aboard the ship *Hopewell* in 1761.[44] Black,[45] Australian aboriginal,[46] and several European[47] kindreds have been described. Sporadic cases also occur. If symptoms first appear after early childhood and there is a negative family history, hereditary nephrogenic diabetes insipidus should be differentiated from acquired vasopressin resistance such as might be found in hypercalcemia, hypokalemia, sickle cell anemia, and various types of chronic renal disease, including amyloidosis[48] and massive hydronephrosis with bladder neck obstruction.[49] In addition there are recent case reports of tumor-associated nephrogenic diabetes insipidus,[50] of nephrogenic diabetes insipidus associated with hyperthyroidism and periodic paralysis,[51] and of diabetes insipidus in association with autosomal dominant hypoparathyroidism.[52] Drug therapy with lithium, declomycin, and amphotericin B may also result in renal-resistant diabetes insipidus.[53,54]

Primary polydipsia is a state of hypotonic polyuria with suppressed AVP levels secondary to excessive fluid intake. It is often psychogenic in origin, the symptoms being less consistent than in patients with central or nephrogenic diabetes insipidus. Increased thirst owing to increased angiotensin levels may occur in patients with renal artery stenosis. Primary polydipsia on an organic basis can also result from hypothalamic disease.[24] Any tendency toward polydipsia can be aggravated by drugs that cause dryness of the mouth.[55] We have investigated two patients who apparently developed primary polydipsia from hypothalamic disease. One patient developed the syndrome soon after a severe blow to the head, and the second patient had thyroid deficiency on a hypothalamic basis together with elevated prolactin levels and thickening of the infundibular stalk. Unlike patients with psychogenic polydipsia,[56] these patients, who apparently had organic polydipsia, had markedly improved symptoms when treated with vasopressin tannate in oil (Pitressin®) or dDAVP. This improvement may be related to the effect of ADH on increasing salivary flow rates and ameliorating thirst in patients with diabetes insipidus.[57]

2. LABORATORY FEATURES

The diagnosis of diabetes insipidus is based on evaluation of the hypothalamo-neurohypophysial system, including both the osmoreceptor mechanism and the ability of AVP to be released in consequence of the activation of this receptor. Stimuli such as nicotine, nausea, and hypotension may release AVP and are useful in attempting to understand the underlying pathophysiological abnormality in individual patients. However, the results are clinically irrelevant. It matters little to the patient with symptomatic diabetes insipidus if we determine that one or all of these nonphysiological or extreme stimuli cause the release of AVP.

The diagnostic procedures that will be discussed in this section were developed in an effort to utilize the known physiological factors that influence vasopressin release as applied to the clinical setting. The appropriate tests, therefore, have to be clinically practical, readily available, rapid in performance, noninjurious to the patient, and preferably inexpensive.

When I first started to work in this field, the laboratory diagnosis of diabetes insipidus was usually based on the presence or absence of a decrease in urine flow rate in patients being infused with hypertonic saline.[58,59] We first reported on the concept of an osmotic threshold for vasopressin release by using 5% saline to raise the plasma osmolality in water-loaded subjects.[13] We found that when a hydrated normal subject was infused with hypertonic saline at a constant rate, there was a linear rise in plasma osmolality with time and that, after an interval depending on the infusion rate, concentration of saline, and initial plasma osmolality, there was an abrupt progressive fall in free water clearance without a change in solute or creatinine excretion. We defined the plasma osmolality at the initiation of antidiuresis under these conditions as the osmotic threshold for vasopressin release and found that it occurred at a mean value of 287.3 mOsm/kg.[13,60] Osmotic threshold studies are conducted by giving the subject a water load, 20 ml/kg, by mouth over a 15- to 20-min period; the water load is maintained with further fluid administration in amounts equal to the volumes of urine passed every 15 min. The patient should remain recumbent between voidings and should have an indwelling needle placed in each forearm, kept patent with dilute (1:1000) heparin solution. When urine volume becomes stable for at least three (preferably five to six) 15-min periods, the patient is given a rapid intravenous infusion of 5% NaCl solution through a forearm needle.

The 5% NaCl solution is administered by infusion pump at 0.05 ml/kg per min. During the saline infusion serum samples are obtained every 15 min for osmolality measurements while the water load is maintained and urine collections are continued every 15 min. This procedure is continued until either 30–45 min after an abrupt reduction in urine flow, indicating that the osmotic threshold has been reached, or until the infusion has continued for more than 2 hr, or until severe headache or discomfort supervenes (whichever comes first).

The free water clearance is calculated on each of the 15-min urine samples before and during the hypertonic saline infusion. When the osmotic threshold has been reached and AVP has been released, there will be an obvious fall in free water clearance by more than 2 SD below the mean free water clearance in the control period. The serum osmolality at the beginning of that 15-min collection period, measured by interpolation on the regression line relating serum osmolality to time, represents the osmotic threshold for AVP release. In normal subjects this will be 284–291 (mean 287.3 ± SD 3.6) mOsm/kg. In patients with primary polydipsia the value is low or normal. In patients with diabetes insipidus an osmotic threshold may occur at an elevated plasma osmolality ("high-set osmoreceptors," "essential hypernatremia") but is usually undetectable even if the serum osmolality is raised to 310–315 mOsm/kg or higher.

Other factors that stimulate AVP release include hypovolemia and hypotension. These mechanisms are much less sensitive in altering hormone release and are considered backup mechanisms; they will not be discussed here in detail. Nonetheless, there is a lower osmotic threshold for vasopressin release when the osmotic stimulus is provided by dehydration than when it is provided by infusion of 5% saline.[61] In contrast to hypovolemia, hypervolemia inhibits the release of AVP and acts to raise the osmotic threshold for release of the hormone.[62]

The first patients with diabetes insipidus whom we investigated had no attainable osmotic threshold, but we soon recognized patients who had elevated osmotic thresholds, and depending on the situation, mainly the sensitivity of the thirst mechanism, could be diagnosed as having either incomplete or partial diabetes insipidus or essential hypernatremia.[63] At the present time we rarely use this test *clinically*, except where there is a problem in differentiating diabetes insipidus from primary polydipsia.

The next procedure that we developed was a dehydration test, which was not based on weight loss or time of water deprivation, but on the premise that normal subjects, regardless of maximal attainable urine osmolality, were limited in their maximum urine osmolality by their renal concentrating mechanism, but that patients with ADH deficiency were limited by the amount of AVP releasable by water deprivation.[64] Since the maximal urinary concentrating capacity varies widely among individuals, it is impossible to distinguish between deficiency and sufficiency of AVP by the absolute level of urinary osmolality attained after specific periods of water deprivation. On the other hand, if after prolonged dehydration, vasopressin administration induces a further rise in urine osmolality, there is a strong implication that vasopressin deficiency exists.

The test that we described is performed by withholding fluids, usually from about 6 AM until the osmolality of successive hourly urine samples increases by less than 30 mOsm/kg, indicating that a plateau of urine concentration has been reached. Constancy of urine osmolality is usually reached by early afternoon. When the plateau is reached, a blood sample is obtained for osmolality and the patient is given aqueous Pitressin, 5 U by subcutaneous injection. Urine is collected at $^1/_2$ hr and 1 hr after this injection for osmolality measurement. Body weights should be recorded at the beginning and end of the dehydration period to determine the percentage of weight lost.

When neurohypophysial reserve is normal, the maximal urinary osmolality after dehydration may be 800–1400 mOsm/kg in robust normal subjects, but may be only 450–800 mOsm/kg in chronically debilitated or malnourished individuals. In all such subjects, urinary osmolality falls slightly or rises by less than 9% after administration of aqueous Pitressin (Figure 2 and Table VI). Patients with primary polydipsia have values similar to those of the debilitated and malnourished subjects. In severe diabetes insipidus, the urinary osmolality reached before the Pitressin injection remains below serum osmolality, while in those patients whose diabetes insipidus is partial or moderately severe, urinary osmolality rises above serum osmolality during dehydration. After the Pitressin injection in subjects whose endogenous vasopressin reserve is normal, urinary osmolality is often lower and is never more than 9% higher than it was immediately before the injection. A Pitressin-induced

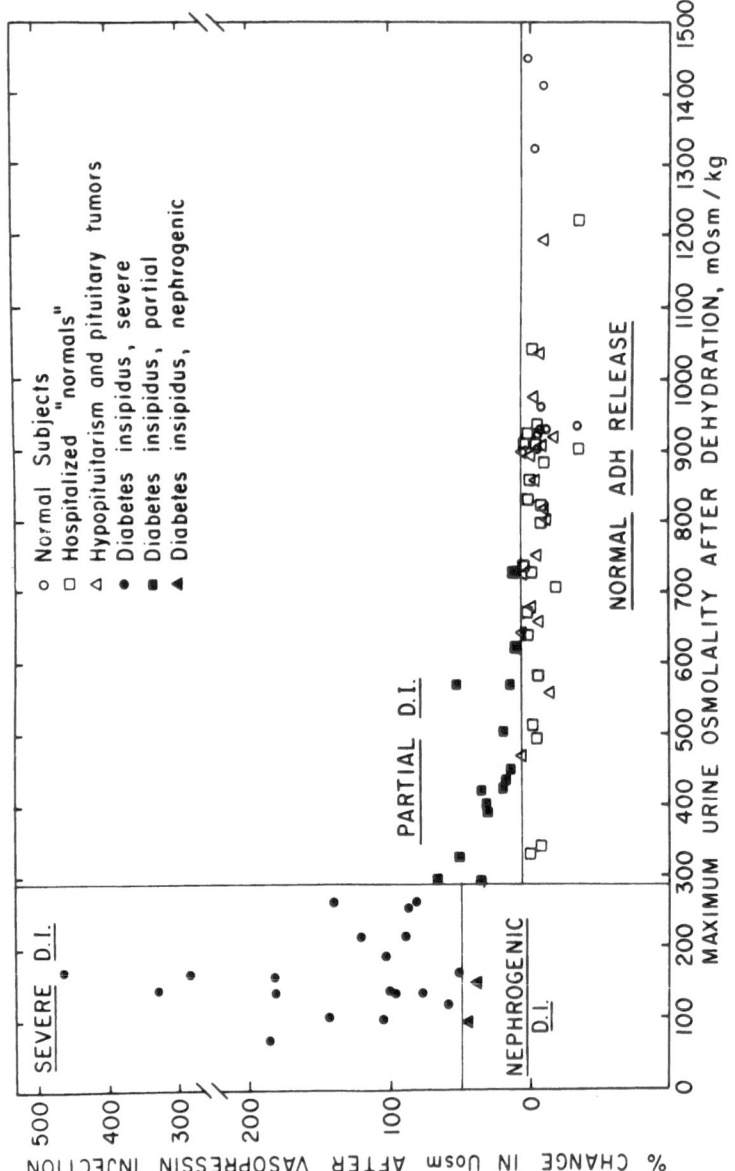

FIGURE 2. Maximum urine osmolality after dehydration plotted against the percentage change in urine osmolality induced by injection of 5 U aqueous Pitressin. (From ref. 64.)

TABLE VI. Interpretation of Dehydration Test

	Maximum Uosm/Posm before pitressin	Maximum Uosm/Posm after pitressin	Uosm increase after pitressin
Normal or primary polydipsia	>1	>1	<9%
Partial ADH[a] deficiency	>1	>1	>9%
Severe ADH deficiency	<1	< or >1	>50%
Nephrogenic diabetes insipidus	<1	<1	<45%

[a] Note that these patients may have severe polyuria.

rise in urinary osmolality of > 50% indicates the presence of vasopressin deficiency or central diabetes insipidus. Patients with nephrogenic diabetes insipidus show a subnormal rise in urinary osmolality after dehydration alone, rarely rising above serum osmolality, and a slight (< 45%) or no rise in urinary osmolality after the Pitressin injection. Patients with primary polydipsia may be so overloaded with fluids that prolonged dehydration may be needed before endogenous AVP is released and urine is concentrated. In these patients, the finding that serum osmolality has not risen above the normal osmotic threshold indicates the need for more prolonged dehydration. This test is simple, generally available, and safe even in patients with profound deficiency of AVP, if severe dehydration is prevented by not allowing body weight to fall by more than 5%.

This test provided much important information about the status of neurohypophysial function in many patients, but it eventually became obvious that the urine osmolality attained during dehydration had to be related carefully to plasma osmolality.[8,63,65,66] For instance, patients were found who had *apparently* normal dehydration tests, but with high plasma osmolalities. Under random conditions, their thirst mechanism might not allow them to get dehydrated enough to concentrate the urine so that under random conditions they would have hypotonic polyuria. If their thirst mechanism was insensitive, they would be classified as having a high-set osmoreceptor or essential hypernatremia. We collected plasma and urine osmolality data during water loading and dehydration and described a normal area indicated by the shaded areas in Figures 3–5.

The plasma versus urine osmolality coordinates can be divided into quadrants (Figure 3). Points that fall in area II (hypertonic urine at an ap-

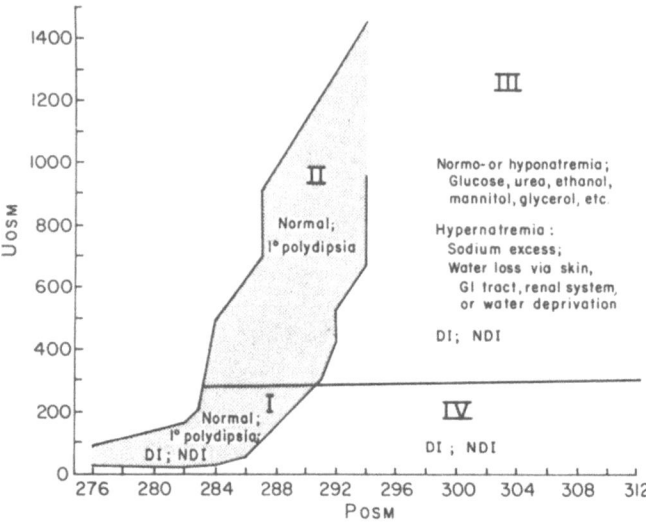

FIGURE 3. Comparison of plasma and urine osmolalities, with data from normal individuals indicated by the shaded area. Coordinates in area II indicate a normal concentrating mechanism, while coordinates in area IV indicate the presence of central or nephrogenic diabetes insipidus. Areas I and IV are indeterminate and patients with such data should be dehydrated or hydrated as detailed in the text.

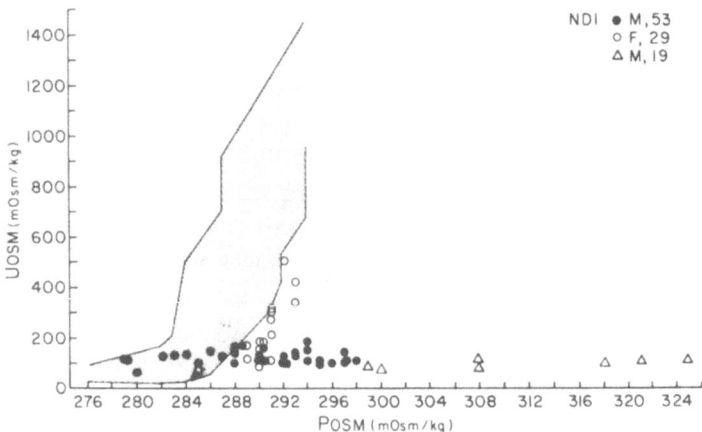

FIGURE 4. Plasma versus urine osmolality coordinates in three patients with nephrogenic diabetes insipidus. Data from normal subjects are included in shaded area.

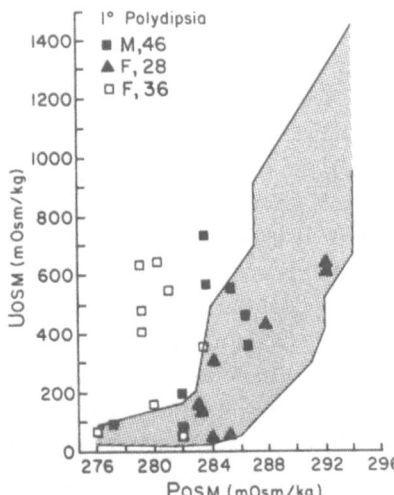

FIGURE 5. Plasma versus urine osmolality coordinates in three patients with primary polydipsia. Shaded area encompasses data obtained in normal subjects.

propriate plasma osmolality) are normal, while points that fall in area IV (hypotonic urine with an elevated plasma osmolality) are abnormal and indicate the presence of central or nephrogenic diabetes insipidus. Points that fall in area I (dilute urine without an elevated plasma osmolality) are indeterminate. To clarify the clinical status of these patients, oral or intravenous fluids should be restricted and urine and plasma osmolality values determined hourly. If the withholding of fluids causes urine versus plasma osmolality coordinates to move into area IV, the patient has diabetes insipidus (if necessary nephrogenic diabetes insipidus can be diagnosed or excluded by the patient's response to administered ADH or by measuring AVP levels in blood or urine (see p. 132). If initial urine and plasma osmolality coordinates are both dilute (area I), dehydration may cause the subsequent points to fall into a normal area where urine is appropriately concentrated in relation to plasma osmolality (area II). This would indicate that the hypotonic polyuria was due to overhydration in a patient with a normal neurohypophysial mechanism. If dehydration causes the urine to become concentrated but only at the expense of an elevated plasma osmolality (area III), the patient probably has an incomplete ADH deficiency. When the pattern becomes clear, the test may be terminated before a plateau in urine osmolality is reached, or alternatively a formal dehydration test may be conducted, as described previously. Plasma or urine levels of AVP usually parallel the urine osmolality (except in patients with nephrogenic diabetes insipidus) and confirm the diagnosis of overhydration or incomplete or severe diabetes insipidus. As noted previously, patients with incomplete or partial diabetes insipidus may have severe polyuria under random conditions if the thirst mechanism is sensitive.

A little-appreciated aspect of the formulation in Figure 3 is that when initial data fall into area III (hypertonicity or hypernatremia with concentrated urine), the gentle forcing of hypotonic fluids will cause subsequent points to fall into areas II or IV, generally allowing a definitive diagnosis to be established. If hydration causes osmolality coordinates to move into area II, the initial hypernatremia was due to water deprivation in a patient with normal neurohypophysial function. If hydration causes the coordinates to move into area IV, the initial hypernatremia was due to a partial deficiency of AVP, a high-set osmoreceptor mechanism, or essential hypernatremia, all of which may be different terminology for the same pathophysiological abnormality.

The use of plasma versus urine osmolality coordinates does not allow the differentiation between central and nephrogenic diabetes insipidus (Figures 3 and 4). However, these two causes of hypotonic polyuria can usually be differentiated by the acute response of urine osmolality to aqueous Pitressin (Figure 2), or by the response to prolonged therapy with Pitressin tannate in oil or dDAVP nasal spray. When a definitive diagnosis is not possible by the use of these methods, measurement of plasma[67,68] or urine AVP[69] allows the diagnosis to be clearly established. In our experience, urinary AVP is normal or supranormal relative to plasma osmolality in patients with nephrogenic diabetes insipidus (Figure 6). In contrast, most patients with central diabetic insipidus have very low levels of urinary AVP in relation to plasma osmolality. Those patients with central diabetes insipidus who have coordinates near the normal area have only very mild polyuria. Figure 7 demonstrates another way of comparing AVP data in patients with central and nephrogenic diabetes insipidus by relating urinary AVP and osmolality. These data demonstrate that under these conditions patients with nephrogenic diabetes insipidus almost always excrete more than 1 mU (2.5 ng) AVP per hour, while patients with central diabetes insipidus excrete less than 1 mU AVP per hour.

The above diagnostic points are usually quite straightforward. However, perhaps 5% of patients have conflicting data. I have never had trouble differentiating central and nephrogenic diabetes insipidus using these criteria, including measurement of AVP levels. Using any technique there will always be a gray area between severe and incomplete central diabetes insipidus. The only clinical problem is whether or not to treat the patient. It may also be difficult to differentiate between incomplete central diabetes insipidus and overhydration (excessive parenteral fluids or primary polydipsia). For example, we recently studied a patient with hypotonic polyuria and normal serum sodium and osmolality who had normal plasma versus urine osmolality coordinates during dehydration (F,28 in Figure 5). She did not increase urine osmolality after Pitressin at the plateau in urine osmolality, but had low AVP levels and increased renal sensitivity to the action of ADH. She was much improved with therapy. She therefore had two criteria for primary polydipsia and two that favored diabetes insipidus. I am uncomfortable in classifying her as having primary polydipsia with a low urinary AVP level in relation to plasma osmolality and with her response to therapy. However, I am also hesitant to say that she has diabetes insipidus with a urine that is normally concentrated in relation to plasma osmolality and with a normal dehydration test. The osmotic threshold test may provide evidence to allow a decision to be made. Response to therapy cannot be used as an ultimate criterion because patients with primary polydipsia on an organic basis may markedly improve with treatment with ADH, the improvement being related to an increased salivary flow rate and amelioration of thirst.[57] In my opinion there is no single ultimate diagnostic standard for the differential diagnosis of the hypotonic polyurias in all cases. The diagnosis has to be based on a combination of factors. Rarely a definitive diagnosis cannot be established.

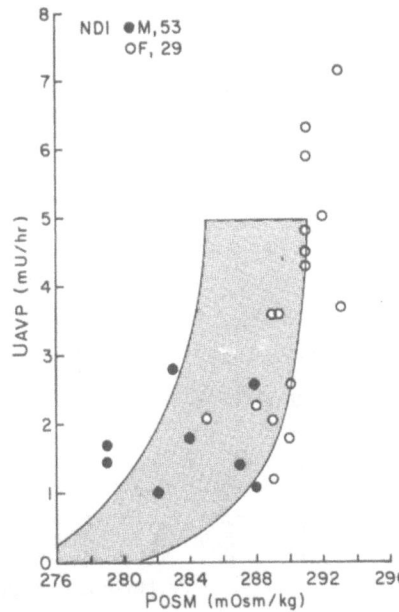

FIGURE 6. Urinary AVP in relation to plasma osmolality in two patients with nephrogenic diabetes insipidus. Shaded area encompasses data obtained in normal subjects.

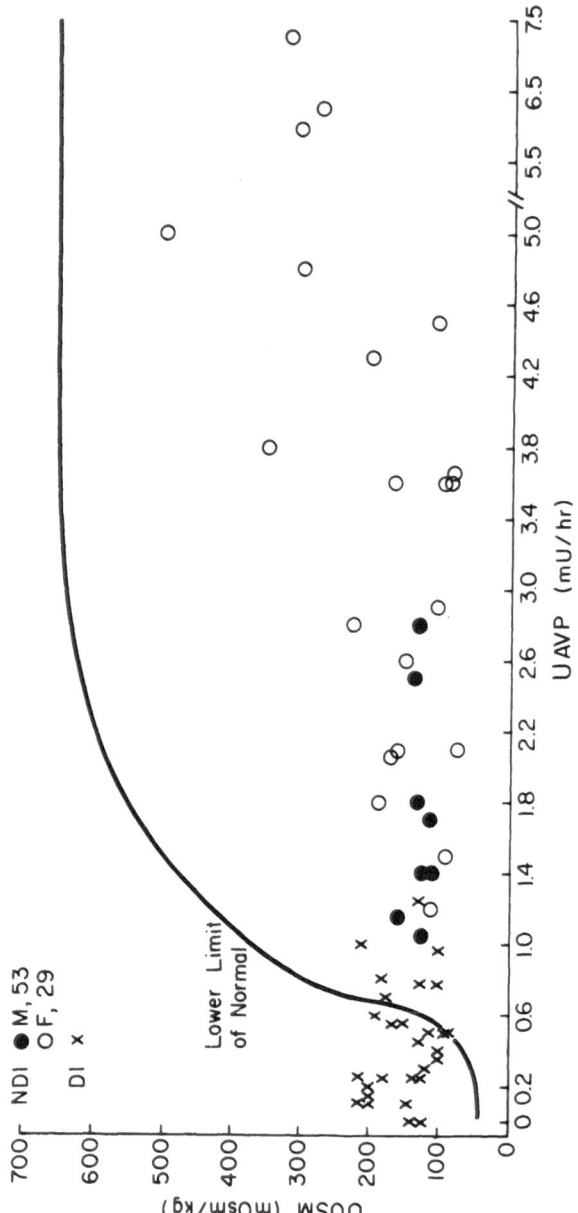

FIGURE 7. Urinary osmolality in relation to urinary AVP in two patients with nephrogenic diabetes insipidus in comparison with data obtained from four patients with central diabetes insipidus, and the lower limit of normal.

3. SUMMARY

Diabetes insipidus is being diagnosed with increasing frequency, particularly the diabetes insipidus caused by blunt head trauma. The term *idiopathic diabetes insipidus* should be reserved for patients who have no other endocrine, neurological, or radiological findings. If any of the latter are present, we should use a term such as *diabetes insipidus, cause to be determined,* and observe the patient closely. The diagnosis of diabetes insipidus can usually be established reliably, quickly, and inexpensively by the use of plasma versus urine osmolality coordinates. The primary role for AVP assays in the differential diagnosis of the hypotonic polyurias is in establishing the presence or absence of nephrogenic diabetes insipidus. Last, it may be difficult and at times even impossible to distinguish central diabetes insipidus from primary polydipsia.

ACKNOWLEDGMENTS. The work on which this chapter is based was supported by Veterans Administration research funds and by Grant RR-229, General Clinical Research Centers Program, Division of Research Resources, National Institutes of Health.

REFERENCES

1. Van Slyck EJ, Jurgensen C, Cargill JW: Diabetes insipidus complicating thrombotic thrombocytopenic purpura. *J Am Med Assoc* 209:768–770, 1969.
2. Veldhuis JD, Hammond JM: Endocrine function after spontaneous infarction of the human pituitary: Report, review and reappraisal. *Endocr Rev* 1:100–107, 1980.
3. Haynes BF, Fauci AS: Diabetes insipidus associated with Wegener's granulomatosis successfully treated with cyclophosphamide. *N Engl J Med* 299:764, 1978.
4. Kelly PM: Systemic blastomycosis with associated diabetes insipidus. *Ann Intern Med* 96:66–67, 1982.
5. Manelfe C, Louvet JP: Computed tomography in diabetes insipidus. *J Comput Assist Tomogr* 3:309–316, 1979.
6. Braverman LE, Mancini JP, and McGoldrick DM: Hereditary idiopathic diabetes insipidus. A case report with autopsy findings. *Ann Intern Med* 63:503–508, 1965.
7. Legros JJ, Crabbe J: Serum neurophysins in familial central diabetes insipidus. *J Clin Endocrinol Metab* 47:1065–1072, 1978.
8. Notman DD, Mortek MA, Moses AM: Permanent diabetes insipidus following head trauma: Observations on ten patients and an approach to diagnosis. *J Trauma* 20:599–602, 1980.
9. Moses AM, Miller M: Osmotic influences on the release of vasopressin, in Greep RO, Astwood EB, Knobil E, et al (eds): *Handbook of Physiology, Endocrinology.* Sect 7, vol IV: *The Pituitary Gland.* Washington, American Physiological Society, 1974, part 1, chap 10, pp 225–242.

IV: *The Pituitary Gland.* Washington, American Physiological Society, 1974, part 1, chap 10, pp 225–242.

10. Quintanilla AP, Delgado-Butron C, Zeballos J: Renal hemodynamics and water excretion in Addison's disease. *Metabolism* 25:419–425, 1976.

11. Boykin J, De Torrente A, Erickson A, et al: Role of plasma vasopressin in impaired water excretion of glucocorticoid deficiency. *J Clin Invest* 62:738–744, 1978.

12. Moses AM, Gabrilove JL, Soffer LJ: Simplified water loading test in hypoadrenocorticism and hypothyroidism. *J Clin Endocrinol Metab* 18:1413–1417, 1958.

13. Aubry RH, Nankin HR, Moses AM, et al: Measurement of the osmotic threshold for vasopressin release in human subjects, and its modification by cortisol. *J Clin Endocrinol Metab* 25:1481–1492, 1965.

14. Savino PJ, Glaser JS, Schatz NJ: Traumatic chiasmal syndrome. *Neurology* 30:963–970, 1980.

15. Barreca T, Perria C, Sannia A, et al: Evaluation of anterior pituitary function in patients with posttraumatic diabetes insipidus. *J Clin Endocrinol Metab* 51:1279–1282, 1980.

16. Machiedo G, Bolanowski PJP, Bauer J, et al: Diabetes insipidus secondary to penetrating thoracic trauma. *Ann Surg* 181:31–34, 1975.

17. Moyson F: Anoxie cérébrale et diabète insipide après inhalation d'un corps étranger chez l'enfant. *Ann Chir Infant* 16:241–248, 1975.

18. Glauser FL: Diabetes insipidus in hypoxemic encephalopathy. *J Am Med Assoc* 235:932–933, 1976.

19. Rothschild M, Shenkman L: Diabetes insipidus following cardiorespiratory arrest. *J Am Med Assoc* 238:620–621, 1977.

20. Taubin H, Matz R: Cerebral edema, diabetes insipidus, and sudden death during the treatment of diabetic ketoacidosis. *Diabetes* 17:108–109, 1968.

21. Parisi JE, Kim RC, Collins GH, et al: Brain death with prolonged somatic survival. *N Engl J Med* 306:14–16, 1982.

22. Winnacker JL, Becker KL, Katz S: Endocrine aspects of sarcoidosis. *N Engl J Med* 278:427–434, 483–492, 1968.

23. Bruning PF, Koster HG, Hekster REM, et al: Sarcoidosis presenting with diabetes insipidus followed by acute cranial nerve syndrome. *Acta Med Scand* 205:441–444, 1979.

24. Stuart CA, Neelon FA, Lebovitz HE: Disordered control of thirst in hypothalamic–pituitary sarcoidosis. *N Engl J Med* 303:1078–1082, 1980.

25. Panitz F, Shinaberger JH: Nephrogenic diabetes insipidus due to sarcoidosis without hypercalcemia. *Ann Intern Med* 62:113–120, 1965.

26. Betkerur U, Shende A, Lanzkowsky P: Acute myeloblastic leukemia presenting with diabetes insipidus. *Am J Med Sci* 273:325–327, 1977.

27. Kornberg A, Zimmerman J, Matzner Y, et al: Acute lymphoblastic leukemia: Association with vasopressin-responsive diabetes insipidus. *Arch Intern Med* 140:1236, 1980.

28. Yap HY, Tashima CK, Blumenschein GR, et al: Diabetes insipidus and breast cancer. *Arch Intern Med* 139:1009–1011, 1979.

29. DeRubertis FR, Michelis MF, Beck N, et al: "Essential" hypernatremia due to ineffective osmotic and intact volume regulation of vasopressin secretion. *J Clin Invest* 50:97–111, 1971.

30. Brezis M, Weiler-Ravell D: Hypernatremia, hypodipsia and partial diabetes insipidus: A model for defective osmoregulation. *Am J Med Sci* 279:37–45, 1980.

31. Kimura T, Matsui K, Ota K, et al: Hypothalamic hypernatremia due to volume-dependent ADH release, and its treatment with carbamazepine and clofibrate. *Tohoku J Exp Med* 127:101–111, 1979.

32. Halter JB, Goldberg AP, Robertson GL, et al: Selective osmoreceptor dysfunction in the syndrome of chronic hypernatremia. *J Clin Endocrinol Metab* 44:609–616, 1977.
33. Mahoney JH, Goodman AD: Hypernatremia due to hypodipsia and elevated threshold for vasopressin release. Effects of treatment with hydrochlorothiazide, chlorpropamide and tolbutamide. *N Engl J Med* 279:1191–1196, 1968.
34. Luciani JC, Conte-Devolx B, Fourcade JC, et al: Chronic hypernatremia, hypovolemia and partial hypopituitarism in sarcoidosis: A case report. *Clin Nephrol* 13:242–247, 1980.
35. Smals AGH, Kloppenborg PWC: Hypernatraemia in human myotonic dystrophy. *Neth J Med* 23:95–103, 1980.
36. Bode HH, Harley BM, Crawford JD: Restoration of normal drinking behavior by chlorpropamide in patients with hypodipsia and diabetes insipidus. *Am J Med* 51:304–313, 1971.
37. Fichman MP, Brooker G: Deficient renal cyclic adenosine 3′,5′monophosphate production in nephrogenic diabetes insipidus. *J Clin Endocrinol Metab* 35:35–47, 1972.
38. Proesmans W, Eggermont E, Vanderschueren-Lodeweyckx M, et al: The effect of exogenous 3′:5′-adenosine monophosphate on urinary output in children with vasopressin-resistant diabetes insipidus. *Pediatr Res* 9:509–512, 1975.
39. Jones NF, Barraclough MA, Barnes N, et al: Nephrogenic diabetes insipidus: Effects of 3′,5′-cyclic-adenosine monophosphate. *Arch Dis Child* 47:794–797, 1972.
40. Sober AJ, Gorden P: Pituitary responsiveness to aqueous vasopressin in patients with congenital vasopressin-resistant diabetes insipidus. *J Clin Endocrinol Metab* 35:924–925, 1972.
41. Valtin H: Genetic models for hypothalamic and nephrogenic diabetes insipidus, in Andreoli TE, Grantham JJ, Rector FC Jr (eds): *Disturbances in Body Fluid Osmolality*. Bethesda, American Physiological Society, 1977, pp 197–215.
42. Dousa TP, Valtin H: Cellular action of antidiuretic hormone in mice with inherited vasopressin-resistant urinary concentrating defects. *J Clin Invest* 54:753–762, 1974.
43. Jackson BA, Edwards RM, Valtin H, et al: Cellular action of vasopressin in medullary tubules of mice with hereditary nephrogenic diabetes insipidus. *J Clin Invest* 66:110–122, 1980.
44. Bode HH, Crawford, JD: Nephrogenic diabetes insipidus in North America: The Hopewell hypothesis. *N Engl J Med* 280:750–754, 1969.
45. Feigin RD, Rimoin DL, Kaufman RL: Nephrogenic diabetes insipidus in a Negro kindred. *Am J Dis Child* 120:64–68, 1970.
46. Schultz P, Lines DR: Nephrogenic diabetes insipidus in an Australian aboriginal kindred. *Humangenetik* 26:79–85, 1975.
47. Buchborn E: Storungen der Harnkonkentrierung, in Mohr L, Staehelin R, Schwiegk H (eds): *Handbuch der Inneren Medizin*. Berlin, Springer-Verlag, 1968, vol 8, part 1, pp 491–673.
48. Ásmundsson P, Snaedal J: Persistent water diuresis in renal amyloidosis. *Scand J Urol Nephrol* 15:77–79, 1981.
49. Ramsey EW, Morrin PAF, Bruce AW: Nephrogenic diabetes insipidus associated with massive hydronephrosis and bladder neck obstruction. *J Urol* 111:225–228, 1974.
50. Feibusch J, Barbosa-Saldivar JL, Bernstein RS, et al: Tumor-associated nephrogenic diabetes insipidus. *Ann Intern Med* 92:797–798, 1980.
51. Bolaños F, Ponce de Léon S, Garcia Ramos G, et al: Hyperthyroidism associated with renal tubular acidosis, nephrocalcinosis, nephrogenic diabetes insipidus and periodic paralysis. *Rev Invest Clin* 33:195–198, 1981.
52. Hunter AGW, Heick H, Poznanski WJ, et al: Autosomal dominant hypoparathyroidism: A proband with concurrent nephrogenic diabetes insipidus. *J Med Genet* 18:431–435, 1981.
53. Singer I, Forrest JN Jr: Drug-induced states of nephrogenic diabetes insipidus. *Kidney Int* 10:82–95, 1976.

54. Barbour GL, Straub KD, O'Neal BL, et al: Vasopressin-resistant nephrogenic diabetes insipidus. A result of amphotericin B therapy. *Arch Intern Med* 139:86–88, 1979.

55. Rao KJ, Miller M, Moses, AM: Water intoxication and thioridazine (Mellaril). *Ann Intern Med* 82:61–63, 1975.

56. Barlow ED, De Wardener HE: Compulsive water drinking. *Q J Med* 28:235–257, 1959.

57. Pasqualini RQ, Codevilla A: Thirst-suppressing (antidipsetic) effect of pitressin in diabetes insipidus. *Acta Endocrinol* 30:37–41, 1959.

58. Hickey RC, Hare K: The renal excretion of chloride and water in diabetes insipidus. *J Clin Invest* 23:768–775, 1944.

59. Carter AC, Robbins J: The use of hypertonic saline infusions in the differential diagnosis of diabetes insipidus and psychogenic polydipsia. *J Clin Endocrinol* 7:753–766, 1947.

60. Moses AM, Streeten DHP: Differentiation of polyuric states by measurement of responses to changes in plasma osmolality induced by hypertonic saline infusions. *Am J Med* 42:368–377, 1967.

61. Moses AM, Miller M: Osmotic threshold for vasopressin release as determined by saline infusion and by dehydration. *Neuroendocrinology* 7:219–226, 1971.

62. Moses AM, Miller M, Streeten DHP: Quantitative influence of blood volume expansion on the osmotic threshold for vasopressin release. *J Clin Endocrinol Metab* 27:655–662, 1967.

63. Miller M, Moses AM: Clinical states due to alteration of ADH release and action, in Moses AM, Share L (eds): *Neurohypophysis.* Basel, S. Karger, 1977, pp 153–166.

64. Miller M, Dalakos T, Moses AM, et al: Recognition of partial defects in antidiuretic hormone secretion. *Ann Intern Med* 73:721–729, 1970.

65. Moses AM, Notman DD: Diabetes insipidus and syndrome of inappropriate antidiuretic hormone secretion (SIADH). *Adv Intern Med* 27:73–100, 1982.

66. Streeten DHP, Moses AM, Miller M: Disorders of the neurohypophysis, in Isselbacher KJ, Adams RD, Braunwald E, et al (eds): *Harrison's Principles of Internal Medicine,* ed 9. New York, McGraw-Hill, 1980, pp 1684–1694.

67. Zerbe RL, Robertson GL: A comparison of plasma vasopressin measurements with a standard indirect test in the differential diagnosis of polyuria. *N Engl J Med* 305:1539–1546, 1981.

68. Kimura T, Matsui K, Sato T, et al: Relationship between plasma osmolality and plasma concentration of antidiuretic hormone in normal subjects, patients with chronic renal disease, and patients with central diabetes insipidus. *Tohoku J Exp Med* 113:77–88, 1974.

69. Miller M, Moses AM: Urinary ADH in polyuric disorders and in inappropriate ADH syndrome. *Ann Intern Med* 77:715–721, 1972.

8

MANAGEMENT OF NEUROGENIC DIABETES INSIPIDUS WITH dDAVP AND OTHER AGENTS

William E. Cobb

In this chapter the treatment of chronic neurogenic diabetes insipidus (DI), the clinical use of vasopressin substitution and nonhormonal antidiuretic agents, and the management of acute DI in hospitalized patients will be reviewed.

1. GENERAL CONSIDERATIONS IN TREATMENT

It is possible with currently available medical therapies to reduce 24-hr urine volume to below 2 liters and to render most patients with neurogenic DI virtually symptom-free. Poorly controlled patients may experience problems in performance at school or work, difficulties in concentration and attention span, tiredness resulting from disturbed sleep, growth retardation, and hydronephrosis. Symptoms can be prevented in almost every patient by replacing the hormone deficiency with vasopressin or one of its analogues; in one half to three quarters of patients effective treatment can be accomplished with nonhormonal agents such as chlorpropamide or a diuretic. The initial

William E. Cobb • Division of Endocrinology and Metabolism, Department of Medicine, Tufts–New England Medical Center Hospital, Boston, Massachusetts 02111.

selection of a drug should be based on an estimate of the extent of vasopressin deficiency; on knowledge of its side effects, with particular reference to the age, habits, and endocrine and cardiovascular status of the patient; and on its cost.

Patients with polyuria in excess of 9 liters/day and urine osmolality after dehydration of less than 100 mOsm/kg have no or very little endogenous vasopressin (complete DI) and will almost always require vasopressin substitution therapy. Conventional neuropophysial preparations either have a short duration of action [aqueous vasopressin, lysine vasopressin (LVP) nasal spray, posterior pituitary snuff] or require intramuscular administration [vasopressin tannate in oil (Pitressin® tannate)], and all have relatively high pressor activity. Newer synthetic analogues of vasopressin are devoid of these problems. 1-Desamino-8-D-arginine vasopressin (dDAVP) is the first and only agent in this class that has been released in the United States. Ease of administration by the intranasal route, excellent control of polyuria, prolonged duration of action, and virtually complete freedom from pressor and other systemic effects are qualities of dDAVP that distinguish it from older therapies used for this condition.[1-9]

Drugs that either potentiate the action of otherwise inadequate quantities of endogenous vasopressin (chlorpropamide) or stimulate its release from the neurophypophysis (clofibrate, carbamazepine), and thiazide diuretics, which impair the renal excretion of free water, may be useful alternatives to vasopressin substitution therapy in selected patients with incomplete vasopressin deficiency. Patients likely to respond to the nonhormonal agents usually have 24-hr urine volume of 8 liters or less per day, and their urine osmolality after dehydration is greater than 100 mOsm/kg. Good control of symptoms and reduction in 24-hr urine volume to 2 liters or less may be possible with nonhormonal agents used singly or in combination in such patients. If control of polyuria with these agents is unsatisfactory or if there is concern over potentially serious reactions to chlorpropamide (hypoglycemia) and carbamazepine (agranulocytosis, aplastic anemia), hormone replacement therapy should be instituted instead.

In the majority of patients with DI, control of polyuria by thiazides, used alone, may be unsatisfactory. Thiazides are most effective in patients who are able to reduce urine volume to 75 ml/hr or less in response to dehydration. In others thiazides have been used successfully in conjunction with other agents to enhance the reduction in urine volume.

2. DRUGS USED TO TREAT NEUROGENIC DIABETES INSIPIDUS

2.1. Conventional Neurohypophysial Preparations

Vasopressin is rapidly inactivated when given orally, so it must be administered parenterally or applied topically to the nasal mucous membranes by dropper, spray, or cotton pledgets. Aqueous vasopressin (20 U/ml) is useful for initiating therapy of DI after surgery or head injury and has been used to supplement the effect of other agents when a rapid but brief antidiuresis is required. The usual dose is 0.1–0.3 ml subcutaneously or intramuscularly. Larger doses (i.e., greater than 5 U or 0.3 ml) may stimulate gastrointestinal smooth muscle and cause nausea, cramping, and diarrhea. Intravenous administration offers no advantage in treating DI and may increase the risk of adverse pressor effects, including constriction of coronary arteries. Angina, myocardial ischemia, and infarction are risks associated with treatment of susceptible patients regardless of the route of administration.

Pitressin tannate was developed to prolong the antidiuretic effect of vasopressin from 6 hr or less to more than 1 day. Good control of polyuria is obtained with 2.5–5 U (0.5–1.0 ml; supplied in 2-ml vials) every 24–48 hr. A major disadvantage is the requirement that it be administered by deep intramuscular injection. Sterile abscess formation and painful injection sites are common problems, and are particularly troublesome in children.[9] Care must be taken to suspend the brown residue at the bottom of the vial, which is the hormone tannate complex, by thorough shaking or heating in warm water. Side effects related to the drug's pressor properties are common problems. Until recently Pitressin was synthesized from vasopressin from bovine neurohypophyses. These extracts contained minor tissue antigens capable of provoking allergic reactions, but the new product, which is made synthetically, should not cause any allergic reactions. Recurrent abdominal pain, uterine cramps, cardiac arrhythmias, and exacerbation of angina are potential side effects of all vasopressin preparations and should be considered prior to the use of this agent.

A short-acting (2–4 hr) nasal spray of synthetic LVP (Diapid®, 50 U/ml) has for the past 20 years been a useful preparation for patients with mild DI[10–12] and has been commonly used to supplement the antidiuretic effect of other agents when a brief antidiuresis is required. Compared to vasopressin it is better tolerated locally, has a slightly longer duration of action, and produces fewer pressor effects. The drug is remarkably well tolerated by most patients, although local and systemic pressor effects may occur.[13] Its major disadvantage is its brief duration of action and the requirement that several doses must be taken throughout the day. Diapid is administered as a nasal spray so that its dose cannot be precisely calculated.

Posterior pituitary snuff is no longer available nor should it have any place in therapy. Local allergic reactions were common with this preparation. The newer agents are better tolerated and permit more precise dosaging.

2.2. dDAVP

dDAVP was synthesized and its activity determined by Zaoral et al. in the mid-1960s.[14] Based on earlier work these investigators correctly predicted that removal of the amino group form N-terminal hemicysteine (position 1) and substitution of D-arginine for L-arginine at position 8 of naturally occurring arginine vasopressin (AVP) would result in a molecule with a long duration of selective antidiuretic action. The key to their success was the discovery that D-arginine substitution at position 8 (DAVP) led to a reduction in pressor activity by nearly three orders of magnitude without notable change in anti-diuretic potency or in duration of action.[15] Their demonstration of a disso-ciation of the two major properties of vasopressin not only made possible the synthesis of a highly specific water-retaining hormone (dDAVP) but also stimulated the development of newer analogues more potent than dDAVP, of others with relatively selective pressor effects, and of analogues that spe-cifically antagonize these actions.

In related studies it was shown that the action of vasopressin could be prolonged by removal of the N-terminal amino group. When both changes are incorporated in a single molecule the resulting peptide dDAVP was shown to have a half-life greater than that of 1-desamino vasopressin and an anti-diuretic potency greater than that of either AVP or DAVP.[15,16]

2.2.1. Comparison of dDAVP with AVP

On a units-per-milligram basis the in vitro antidiuretic activity of dDAVP is about 2.5–3 times that of AVP, but dDAVP has only a small fraction

TABLE I. Comparison of the Biological Activities of AVP
and dDAVP

	AVP	dDAVP
Activities (1 U/mg)		
Antidiuretic	400	1000[a]
Pressor	400	0.27
AD/P	1	2000
Duration of effect (hr)	1–6	6–20
Disappearance half-life	24	7.8 (1st exponential)
(minutes after		75.5 (2nd exponential)
intravenous injection)		
Effect on adrenocorticotropic	↑	No change
hormone secretion		

[a] Burns assay in trained unanesthetized rats. Antidiuretic activities in other assays
may be several times greater.

(about 1/750th) of the pressor activity. The antidiuretic specificity (AD/P),
which is the ratio of antidiuretic to pressor activity, takes both properties into
account; for dDAVP the AD/P exceeds 2000 compared to an AD/P of 1 for
AVP.[16] The duration of action in the dosage range used in humans ranges
from 6 (occasionally less) to 20 hr or more for dDAVP, as compared to 1–6
hr for the antidiuretic equivalent of AVP. The clinical importance of these
properties is that the antidiuretic action of dDAVP is sufficiently prolonged
to require administration of the drug only twice daily in most patients and
that the usually effective antidiuretic doses are below the threshold level for
a pressor response or for stimulation of nonvascular smooth muscle. Con-
sequently, side effects related to vasoconstriction or to intestinal, bladder,
and uterine stimulation, common with AVP, do not occur (or do so only
rarely at high doses) with dDAVP. These differences and others are summarized in Table I.

2.2.2. Renal Response to dDAVP

Urine volume begins to fall and osmolality to increase within 1 hr after
intranasal or intravenous dDAVP. The peak response of urine osmolality is
probably no greater with dDAVP than with AVP[17] because urine concentration
is limited by counter current forces that determine the medullary interstitial
gradient and not by tubular responsiveness.[18] However, study of the renal

tubular response in vitro, using isolated rat renal medulla, suggests that the cellular action of dDAVP is more potent than that of AVP. In this system maximum adenyl cyclase activity is increased threefold and cyclic AMP (cAMP) accumulation tenfold by dDAVP, relative to AVP.[17] Because the peak (as well as submaximal) response to dDAVP was increased and because there was no evidence for increased receptor binding of dDAVP, this study suggests that the greater potency of dDAVP is due to enhanced postreceptor stimulation of adenyl cyclase. The relative importance of this effect and whether it occurs at all in humans have not been determined. It is possible that the peak urine osmolality after dDAVP may be maintained longer because of a more prolonged elevation of cAMP. More important clinically is its prolonged effect owing to resistance to enzymatic degradation[3,19] (see Section 2.2.3).

The renal tubular response to dDAVP, like that to AVP, may be under inhibitory control by prostaglandins. The vasopressin-deficient Brattleboro rat excretes large quantities of prostaglandin E_2 (PGE_2) in urine after AVP or dDAVP treatment[20] (PGE_2 levels before treatment are very low in Brattleboro rats).[21] However, the site of dDAVP-stimulated prostaglandin synthesis has not been established. Unlike AVP, dDAVP does not exert an effect on PGE_2 synthesis in vitro in rat renal medullary cells.[22] Zusman has suggested that stimulation of PGE_2 by dDAVP may take place in collecting duct epithelium, although the site has not been directly studied.[23] In humans indirect support for an inhibitory role of prostaglandins on the renal response to dDAVP comes from a study by Moses et al., who demonstrated that indomethacin, an inhibitor of prostaglandin synthesis, increases the peak urine osmolality that occurs in response to low doses of subcutaneous dDAVP.[24] Unlike the Brattleboro rat, humans do not increase the urinary excretion of PGE_2 after dDAVP.[25] PGE_2 excretion in man is dependent on urine flow rate and not on vasopressin status or state of hydration, so that treatment of humans with dDAVP actually leads to a fall in urinary PGE_2.[25]

2.2.3. Factors Determining the Response to dDAVP

A dose–response relationship has been shown to exist over the entire range of doses of dDAVP used in clinical practice.[19,26] However, whether the response is expressed as a function either of the peak reduction in urine flow or of the antidiuretic effect over a period of time, it correlates most closely with the log dose, so that the increment in antidiuretic effectiveness actually declines per unit increase in dose. This may become a matter of practical importance when cost becomes a factor in treatment (see Section 2.2.4a).

After a single 20-μg intranasal dose of dDAVP, urine volume remains below 75 cc/hr and osmolality above 400 mOsm/kg for 5–21 hr.[25] The duration of response is related directly to the plasma half-life of dDAVP, and the wide variation in duration of response to differences among individual subjects in its absorption from nasal mucosa and in its disappearance from blood.[17] In a group of six patients with neurogenic DI Seif et al. determined that the half-life of disappearance ranged from 24 min to 4 hr and showed the strong correlation of blood level with duration of antidiuresis. Peak plasma levels of dDAVP were observed as early as 30 min to as long as 4 hr after intranasal administration, ranged more than fourfold from a low of 21 to a high of 96 pg/ml, and far exceeded the minimum concentration required for a full effect; the maximum renal response persisted long after plasma dDAVP fell below 6 pg/ml, which is the lowest concentration measured in their radioimmunoassay.[17] Pullan et al. have also demonstrated a correlation between the duration of action of dDAVP and its plasma half-life, which they determined to be 89–153 min.[27]

While it is by no means certain that increased biochemical stability is the only explanation for the prolonged half-life of dDAVP, differences in its rate of disappearance from blood and in its in vitro rate of degradation relative to LVP and AVP, which have a much shorter duration of action, have been observed. After intravenous administration both the first and second exponential half-lives of dDAVP (7.8 and 75.5 min) exceeded those of LVP (2.5 and 14.5 min)[3]; from other work the half-life of AVP has been estimated to be 24 min.[28] Human pregnancy plasma contains high levels of an aminopeptidase that cleaves vasopressin at the hemicysteine residue in position 1. However, in the nonpregnant state plasma degradative enzymes do not play an important role in vasopressin metabolism. Under normal conditions C-terminal dipeptide cleavage in the kidney seems to be the major route of AVP inactivation[29]; enzymatic activity leading to vasopressin degradation is also present in the liver, diencephalon, and other organs.[30] It has also been suggested that differences in physicochemical properties between AVP and dDAVP may explain the longer half-life of dDAVP.[15] dDAVP has a more compact three-dimensional size and is more lipophilic than AVP, and for these reasons it may be reabsorbed to a greater extent by renal tubular cells and may be distributed more widely so that its glomerular clearance is reduced. The duration of response to dDAVP varies not only between patients[31,32] but also at different times in individuals receiving the same dose of intranasal dDAVP.[9,19,33,34] Changes in local factors or minor variations in administration technique may alter the rate or fraction of drug absorbed from the nasal mucosa, and in one reported case the renal tubular response, expressed as peak urine osmolality, actually increased as the duration of response became shorter.[33] In a small number of patients a permanent loss or reduction of effectiveness occurs.[9,19,33] Cort et al. have suggested that repeated administration of dDAVP may in some way enhance its own degradation,[19] but whether it is a change in degradation rate or a change in other factor(s) involved in the metabolic clearance of dDAVP that occurs is not known. No evidence for antibody-mediated destruction of dDAVP[9] or for "antivasopressin" activity[19] has been found in patients who have developed "resistance" to the antidiuretic effect of dDAVP.

2.2.4. Clinical Use of dDAVP in Neurogenic DI

dDAVP has been administered intranasally to treat diabetes insipidus in a wide variety of clinical situations (Table II). Special problems may arise that are related to the intranasal mode of administration or to the use of

TABLE II. Clinical Situations in Which Intranasal dDAVP Has Been Used to Manage Neurogenic Diabetes Insipidus

A. Chronic treatment in adults and children
B. Acute diabetes insipidus
   1. Postoperative
      a. Craniotomy
      b. Transsphenoidal surgery[a]
   2. Anoxic encephalopathy
   3. Intraventricular hemorrhage in infants
C. Pregnancy
D. Essential hypernatremia and other conditions
   in which there is an impairment of thirst

[a] Intranasal dDAVP has not been used when the nose is occluded with packing.

vasopressin substitution therapies in general. Intranasal dDAVP cannot be administered to patients in the very early postoperative period following transsphenoidal surgery because of the presence of nasal packing. The intravenous or subcutaneous preparations now used in Europe, but presently unavailable in the United States, are useful in this setting. Intranasal dDAVP is absorbed from the nasal mucosa as early as 24 hr after removal of packing. Treatment of unconscious patients or infants can be achieved by attaching the catheter containing liquid dDAVP to a small air-filled syringe for delivery of the solution into the nasal cavity. The risk of causing hyponatremia is greatest in infants or in adults with depressed consciousness who cannot control the volume of water intake themselves, and in patients with impaired thirst. Individuals concurrently receiving thiazides, chlorpropamide, or antiinflammatory nonsteroidal prostaglandin synthesis inhibitors, all of which have a predominantly renal mechanism of action, and patients receiving neuroleptics, which may enhance drinking behavior, are also at risk of developing hyponatremia during treatment with dDAVP or other vasopressin substitution therapies.

Special mention should be made of the use of dDAVP in pregnancy. At least 25 women[35] are known to have received the drug during pregnancy without ill effect on the patient or fetus.[34,36,37] While other vasopressin substitution therapies commonly lose much of their effectiveness during pregnancy,[36,38] this does not seem to be true of dDAVP treatment. Burrow has reported that dDAVP is either not present at all or present in very small amounts[37] in the breast milk of women under treatment, suggesting that breast-feeding may be permitted without concern that the drug will be passed on to the child.

2.2.4a. Dosage and Administration. In adults good control of neurogenic DI can usually be achieved with twice-daily nasal insufflation of dDAVP, although three or more doses or, rarely, only a single daily dose may be needed. Of 40 patients treated in our clinic (Table III) only two require more than 30 μg per day, 70% require 20 μg or less daily, and 25% need only 10 μg or less per day. Children seem to require slightly lower doses than adults,[4,5,7] and infants may sometimes be adequately controlled at a fraction of the adult dose.[39]

The amount required on a daily basis does not correlate with the severity of symptoms, or with the volume or osmolality of 24-hr urine collections prior to treatment, but may vary widely in some patients depending on the

TABLE III. The Clinical Features of 40 Patients
before Treatment with dDAVP

Age	5–58 years
Duration	2 months to 6 years
Urine volume (before treatment)	2.5–25 liters per 24 hr
Diagnosis	
Postsurgical	22
Empty sella	2
Hypothalamic disease	8
Idiopathic	8

chosen frequency of administration.[9] It is important to establish the smallest dose that results in comfort for the patient because dDAVP is expensive (1 μg of dDAVP costs approximately $0.11 based on the average wholesale cost to retail pharmacies in December 1983). Its cost in relation to that of other agents is shown in Table IV.

Treatment can be started at home by establishing, as the first objective, a dose, taken at bedtime, that allows the patient to sleep uninterrupted by the need to urinate. We begin with 2.5 μg and increase by 2.5-μg increments until this objective is reached. While determining the optimal nighttime dose we instruct the patients to take the same or a smaller dose during the day, although we ask them first to wait until the effect of the previous night's dose has worn off, so that an approximation of its duration of effect can be made. When the evening dose has been determined the daytime dose is then taken shortly before the evening dose loses it effect, and it is adjusted to provide satisfactory control of polyuria throughout the day. The usual result is a

TABLE IV. Cost of the Agents Most Often Used to Treat
Neurogenic Diabetes Insipidus

Drug	Dose	Approximate wholesale cost per month
1. dDAVP	10 μg bid	$66.00
2. Pitressin tannate	5 units qod	18.50[a]
3. Hydrochlorothiazide	50 mg bid	2.10
4. Clofibrate	500 mg qid	13.60
5. Carbamazepine	200 mg tid	19.75
6. Chlorpropamide	250 mg qd	7.83

[a] Does not include cost of syringes and needles.

convenient twice-daily dosage schedule, with a daytime dose that is slightly greater than that required at bedtime. If it becomes necessary to raise the daytime dose to more than 1.5–2 times the bedtime dose, a more frequent administration schedule should be considered. As a practical matter, once a dose that provides 8 or more hr of good control has been determined, attempts to prolong the duration of antidiuresis by increasing the size of a single dose may result in a much greater consumption of dDAVP than the use of smaller, divided doses.

An appreciation of this phenomenon may be had by assuming that the biologic half-life of dDAVP is approximately the same as its disappearance half-life in plasma,* and by assuming that the peak plasma level will increase in direct proportion to the increase in dose. A doubling of dose will therefore raise the peak plasma level by 100% and prolong the duration of effect by one half-life; another doubling of dose (four times original dose) will increase the peak level to four times its original value but will result in a prolongation of effect of only two half lives, and so on. If we assume an elimination half-life for dDAVP of 75 min[3] (see Section 2.3.3), consider the dose of dDAVP that would be required to increase the duration of antidiuretic effect to 12 hr in a patient who is controlled for 8 hr by a 5-μg dose. An increase in duration of response by 4 hr represents more than three half-lives (225 min) and would require three progressive doublings of dosage, or a theoretical dose that exceeds 40 μg. If instead a repeat 5-μg dose were taken after 8 hr, the patient could be controlled for 16 hr by as little as 10 μg dDAVP. The difference expressed in cost savings is greater than $75/month.

2.2.4b. Changes in Response during Treatment. The most common problem that occurs during long-term treatment of patients with dDAVP is a reduction in its antidiuretic efficacy. When serial 24-hr urine collections for volume and osmolality are examined in the same patient, it becomes apparent that the few patients who complain of a change in response lie at the extreme end of a phenomenon that occurs in all patients.[9] Eight patients (20%) in our series have noted a temporary change in response on more than four occasions. Six of these are women and in three the loss of effect was noticeable during the initial 3–4 days of menstruation; it may be that the lower level of estrogen

---

*The basis for this assumption is the correlation between biologic effect and disappearance half-life; inspection of the renal response, expressed as urine flow rate or osmolality, versus time with increasing doses of dDAVP also indicates that the assumption is a reasonable one.

in the early follicular phase results in a reduction in blood flow to nasal mucous membranes, or in some other way retards the absorption of dDAVP. Five patients have noticed reduced effectiveness during times of increased physical activity. Upper airway congestion and emotional stress have also been reported as factors that interfere with drug effect.[34] Whether factors exist that cause temporary changes in the metabolic clearance of dDAVP is not known. Water loading has been reported to enhance the renal clearance of endogenous AVP.[40]

Rarely a permanent change in response occurs.[9,20,21] Such patients are most likely examples of individuals described by Rado as rapid metabolizers of dDAVP and whom he has shown have a history of shortened response to agents such as clofibrate and chlorpropamide that depend on endogenous levels of vasopressin.[41] Possible approaches to manage such patients include the addition of agents that potentiate the renal tubular response to vasopressin,[42] of thiazide diuretics that act by a renal mechanism independent of vasopressin, or the use of more potent, longer-acting analogues, such as deamino-(4-valine, 8-D-arginine)-vasopressin (dVDAVP)[19,43] which are not yet available in the United States. We have found that hydrochlorothiazide restored water balance to normal in two resistant patients who did not benefit from clofibrate. A third patient in our group discontinued dDAVP entirely and is satisfactorily controlled with Pitressin tannate.

2.2.4c. Side Effects and Adverse Reactions to dDAVP. The only side effect observed in our patients is headache (2 males). In one a change to smaller, more frequent doses eliminated the problem, and in the other headache became a problem only as the patient acquired resistance to the antidiuretic effect of dDAVP and exceeded a total daily dose of 50 μg. Although its mechanism is unclear, headache has been reported in other studies in which high doses of dDAVP were used. We believe that it may be due to a local nasal effect since both of our patients had infrequent headaches during previous treatment with Pitressin tannate. Other side effects rarely reported include transient nasal congestion, rhinitis, flushing, abdominal cramps, vulvar pain, sweating, and uneasiness at micturition.[34] Small increases in blood pressure have occurred at doses of 40 μg or more.[19] No idiosyncratic or long-term adverse effects on the hematopoietic system, on liver and kidney function, or on the function of other organs have been reported. Allergies and other adverse immunologic reactions have not occurred.

2.3. Nonhormonal Agents

In the past 25 years a remarkable number of drugs developed for other medical uses have been found to have potent antidiuretic properties. Many of these have been used to probe the mechanism of vasopressin secretion and action and some have become popular in the treatment of DI. Thiazide diuretics, chlorpropamide, carbamazepine, and clofibrate are the best known and most widely used agents, although acetaminophen, an over-the-counter analgesic, has significant antidiuretic activity and might well have taken a place in the therapeutic armamentarium of endocrinologists had its clinical effects been pursued with more vigor.[44,45] Tolbutamide, the first widely used oral sulfonylurea, has antidiuretic properties but is too weak an agent for satisfactory control of DI, and cyclophosphamide, an antimetabolite, is too toxic. The most recent class of drugs to receive attention is the nonsteroidal antiinflammatory agents, in particular indomethacin, which is only the second drug (thiazides being the first) shown to have an antidiuretic effect in patients with nephrogenic DI.[46] Most clinicians currently prefer to use specific vasopressin analogues such as dDAVP in managing chronic DI, but it should not be forgotten that the oral agents may be highly effective low-cost alternatives in selected patients.

2.3.1. Chlorpropamide

Chlorpropamide is an oral sulfonylurea used to treat diabetes mellitus that was first shown to have a beneficial antidiuretic effect by Arduino et al. when they observed a reduction in nonglycosuric polyuria during the treatment of a patient who suffered from both diabetes mellitus and DI.[47] Although it was established in their work and by others[48] that the antidiuresis produced by chlorpropamide resembled that of vasopressin in all respects, it soon became apparent that chlorpropamide alone is inactive[49–51] and that its major action is to enhance the antidiuretic effect of vasopressin by potentiating the vasopressin-stimulated rise in cAMP.[52] In early studies the mechanism of the chlorpropamide effect was thought to be impaired degradation of cAMP by phosphodiesterase,[52–54] but Moses et al. have recently shown that increased synthesis of cAMP is the probable mechanism,[55] and have proposed that chlorpropamide has its effect directly on the vasopressin receptor, where it augments the response to AVP, or to analogues such as dDAVP.[56] Chlorpropamide has also been shown to inhibit vasopressin-stimulated PGE_2 synthesis,[57] suggesting that its antidiuretic effect may be due in part to reduced feedback inhibition of vasopressin action by PGE_2. However, under different experimental conditions chlorpropamide has been shown to enhance vasopressin-stimulated PGE_2 synthesis, suggesting that suppression of PGE_2-mediated feedback inhibition of vasopressin action is probably not an important mechanism for the antidiuretic effect of chlorpropamide.[56] That chlorpropamide may directly stimulate vasopressin secretion has been suggested by studies that show a rise in urine vasopressin levels after chlorpropamide administration.[49] However, radioimmunoassay determinations of both AVP and neurophysin concentrations in plasma have not confirmed a rise after chlorpropamide, and have given rise to doubt that chlorpropamide directly stimulates neurohypophysial secretion.[58]

Approximately half of all patients with neurogenic DI are well controlled, i.e., have a urine volume of 2 liters or less per day at a daily dose of 50–500 mg chlorpropamide.[53,59] Another 25–30% show a definite reduction in urine volume, but symptomatic polyuria persists. The addition of another nonhormonal agent, such as a thiazide diuretic[60] or carbamazepine,[61] results in satisfactory control of polyuria in a high percentage of patients who have only a partial response to chlorpropamide alone. The use of other nonhormonal drugs in combination with chlorpropamide is also of value when dose-related side effects occur with a single agent.[62] Treatment with two drugs permits lower doses of each to be used, and with a better combined effect than is seen with either agent used alone.

Several reports have suggested that chlorpropamide is of particular value in the syndrome of DI associated with absent or diminished thirst.[63,64] These patients demonstrate hypernatremia with minimal or no volume deficiency, intact renal tubular responsiveness to vasopressin, and impaired vasopressin response to osmotic stimuli but normal response to volume depletion.[65] They behave as though osmoreceptor control of thirst and vasopressin secretion has been resent to a higher threshold. Many such patients treated with chlorpropamide have shown a reduction in plasma osmolality and urine volume and a rise in urine osmolality, suggesting that chlorpropamide activates the osmoreceptor response to osmotic stimuli.

Adverse Effects.   Chlorpropamide should be used cautiously in children and adults with hypopituitarism because profound hypoglycemia may develop.[59] Patients with intact anterior pituitaries may also develop hypoglycemia, but the reactions are not likely to be as severe or life-threatening as in the group with impaired function. The prolonged half-life of chlorpropamide may permit the development of water intoxication in patients who consume large amounts of alcohol or other beverages[59]; it should probably not be prescribed to patients whose business or social activities include frequent entertaining or drinking. Alcohol ingestion may also increase the likelihood of hypoglycemia or result in symptoms resembling an Antabuse® reaction. Its effect may be substantially prolonged in renal failure and in patients with congestive heart failure.

2.3.2. Clofibrate

Clofibrate is a lipid-lowering drug that has a significant antidiuretic effect in mild to moderately severe DI.[66] It is believed to act by facilitating the neurohypophysial secretion of endogenous vasopressin because the urinary excretion of vasopressin rises in fully hydrated normal subjects who are given the drug.[66] Clofibrate in doses that are ineffective alone has been shown to prolong the effect of dDAVP in patients with DI,[42] suggesting that it may also have an action on renal tubular cells or slow the degradation of dDAVP. The drug is ineffective in severe DI and in nephrogenic DI,[67] which suggests that it has no intrinsic antidiuretic activity.

Clofibrate in a dose of 2 g daily may reduce urine volume by 50% or more in selected patients with DI. Used alone it is probably less effective than chlorpropamide, but some patients have been shown to benefit by the use of both drugs in combination, at doses lower than would be expected to have an effect if either were used alone.[68]

Side Effects and Adverse Reactions. The most common side effects are gastrointestinal (nausea, vomiting, dyspepsia, flatulence, and diarrhea) and usually disappear with continued treatment. Weight gain (not due to a positive water balance), small reversible elevations in serum transaminase levels, and a rise in skeletal muscle creatine phosphokinase sometimes accompanied by frank myositis may occur. Clofibrate displaces the binding of acidic drugs from plasma proteins so that the dosage of coumarin anticoagulants, diphenylhydantoin, and tolbutamide should be reduced in patients beginning treatment with clofibrate. Its use in pregnancy has not been studied and the drug is excreted in breast milk.

There are no reports of its long-term safe use in DI, so that treated patients should be followed closely for adverse effects.

2.3.3. Carbamazepine

Carbamazepine is a tricyclic anticonvulsant that is thought to act by stimulating the neurohypophysial secretion of vasopressin.[69] Although a rise in plasma vasopressin has been shown by bioassay, no change in radioimmunoassayable vasopressin levels has been found after carbamazepine administration, which raises questions about its exact mechanism of action in DI.[70] The drug has no intrinsic antidiuretic activity and does not enhance the effects of vasopressin in animals.

Carbamazepine at a dose of 400–600 mg/day is effective alone or may result in a synergistic antidiuretic effect along with chlorpropamide.[63]

Side Effects and Adverse Reactions. A variety of neurologic reactions resembling those that occur with the chemically related tricyclic antidepressants may occur, especially in the early treatment period. These include lightheadedness, ataxia, dry mouth, constipation, and urinary retention. Severe hypersensitivity dermatologic reactions occur occasionally. Leukopenia, eosinophilia, and, rarely, aplastic anemia, agranulocytosis, or thrombocytopenia may develop in treated patients. These effects are reversible but may cause death if not promptly recognized. Concern over these reactions and the availability of safer alternative treatments have resulted in infrequent use of carbamazepine in DI.

2.3.4. Thiazide Diuretics

Crawford and Kennedy, in 1959, were the first to report on the usefulness of thiazide diuretics in the treatment of neurogenic DI and were able to establish that the effect of thiazides was independent of vasopressin action in the kidney by demonstrating effectiveness in patients with nephrogenic DI.[72] Since then thiazides have become the mainstay of treatment of nephrogenic

DI and have been widely used in combination with other agents, and occasionally alone, to treat neurogenic DI. The mechanism of action of thiazides is complex. Their main effect is to inhibit (sodium) chloride reabsorption in the distal tubule, which accounts for the impairment in urinary dilution that occurs with their use.[73] Prolonged administration creates a negative salt balance, a reduction in extracellular fluid volume, and a reduced glomerular filtration rate.[74] The latter effects seem to be important for its usefulness as an antidiuretic agent because the antidiuretic effect is abolished if enough sodium chloride is ingested to prevent a negative salt balance and reduction in extracellular volume.

Hydrochlorothiazide, 25–100 mg daily, may be effective as a sole treatment in patients with mild symptoms. An important limitation of thiazides is that the urine of patients with moderate to severe vasopressin deficiency never becomes hypertonic, although it may approach isotonicity with plasma. However, when used in conjunction with nonhormonal agents or with vasopressin substitution therapies, thiazides may result in further amelioration of symptoms and at considerably lower cost to patients than the addition of other agents.

3. MANAGEMENT OF ACUTE NEUROGENIC DIABETES INSIPIDUS

When DI develops in an acutely ill medical patient or following neurosurgery for hypothalamic and pituitary tumors, water loss may approach 1200–1500 cc/hr in extreme cases. If the patient is unconscious or unable to communicate, or if urine output is not carefully monitored by the hospital staff, complications from dehydration may occur rapidly. Accurate diagnosis and prompt treatment of the condition are necessary to avoid the development of grave alterations in solute and water balance.

3.1. Pathogenesis

The successful management of acute DI, especially in the patient recovering from neurosurgery or trauma, requires an appreciation and understanding of the triphasic pattern of alteration in vasopressin secretion that can occur in this setting.[75,76] The changes that develop are similar to those first observed by Fisher et al. in 1938 following experimental injury to the neurohypophysial system of the cat.[77] After damage to the supraotic and paraventricular nuclei the initial effect is the immediate development of polyuria and polydipsia. This first or "transient" phase lasts from hours to as long as 7 days and is the result of elimination of neural impulses regulating hormone secretion consequent to sudden injury to axons and nerve cell bodies. Clinically, any manipulation or disease process that directly damages the hypothalamus or the high infundibular stalk and causes a 90% or greater interruption in axoplasmic flow in the median eminence and below may elicit this response. The second phase ("interphase") is characterized by a progressive reduction in urine volume toward baseline, and the patient (or animal) may appear normal. The normal appearance is misleading because in this phase vasopressin is released in an unregulated fashion from injured axons and from posterior pituitary stores, as these structures undergo degeneration.[78] If the posterior pituitary is deliberately removed prior to damaging the hypothalamus, permanent DI develops without an interphase.[79] During the interphase the ability of patients to excrete a water load is limited by the release of vasopressin; excretion of an inappropriately concentrated urine of low volume may persist for several days and, if the administration of water is not curtailed, hyponatremia and symptoms of water intoxication may develop. The third component of the classic response is the reappearance of polyuria, which occurs when the stores of vasopressin are depleted and is thought to represent irreversible DI. However, occasional patients with apparent "permanent DI" may, after months or even years, recover from their injury and begin to secrete vasopressin in amounts adequate for normal water homeostasis. Hence one should always evaluate the necessity for therapy at intervals for several years after injury.

Clinically, two additional patterns of response may be seen after surgery.[80] Temporary polyuria followed by a return to normal is the most common type, especially after less extensive surgery of the stalk region such as the transsphenoidal removal of a microadenoma. This brief aberration is probably due to transient interruption of neurohypophysial secretion secondary to alterations in blood flow and the development of local edema following manipulation of the infundibular stalk. In the second type permanent DI develops without an interphase. This is more likely to occur after removal of large pituitary or hypothalamic tumors and resembles the Fisher model described above, in which the pituitary was removed before experimental damage to the supraoptic and paraventricular nuclei.

3.2. Evaluation and Treatment[80,81]

Whenever the diagnosis of DI is considered in the differential diagnosis of polyuria of abrupt onset, treatment should be withheld until the characteristic laboratory changes are present (see Chapter 7). The diagnosis of DI is confirmed by demonstrating an abnormally high serum osmolality (>295 mOsm/kg) and an inappropriately dilute urine (<300 mOsm/kg). If the serum osmolality is normal, the diuresis should be allowed to continue until a state of mild serum hyperosmolality is achieved, thus avoiding an erroneous diagnosis of DI in a patient undergoing a water diuresis because of overhydration. Overhydration is particularly likely to occur in surgical patients, and diuresis of the excess fluid may not follow until several hours postoperatively. Vasopressin secretion is part of the reason for postoperative oliguria[82]; preoperative narcotics and barbiturates may stimulate vasopressin release by a central mechanism. The effect may be amplified by anesthetic agents, which prevent reflex inhibition of vasopressin secretion by inhibiting the activity of volume-sensitive stretch receptors in the vascular system. Patients undergoing a water diuresis will have a low or normal serum osmolality, a low urine osmolality and a low or normal serum sodium concentration. A normal or high serum and high urine osmolality suggest an osmotic diuresis, most often due to osmotic agents such as mannitol (used to reduce brain swelling) or to glycosuria in a diabetic patient. The latter situation may be easily missed in the mild diet-controlled diabetic who manifests glycosuria only on exposure to high-dose steroids and the stress of surgery. Serum sodium concentration is of particular value in the setting of an osmotic diuresis because dilution of extracellular fluid by the osmotically active agent may result in hyponatremia. Osmotic diuresis may also occur in chronic renal failure.

Corticosteroids and diphenylhydantoin, drugs that have a minor inhibitory effect on ADH release in normals,[83] may aggravate the manifestations of DI in patients with compromised ADH reverse. Aubry et al.[84] reported that pretreatment of human subjects with hydrocortisone could raise the osmotic threshold for ADH release during normal saline infusion. Streeten et al.[85] have provided more direct support for an effect of steroids on osmore-

ceptor function by demonstrating that cortisol injected directly into the supraoptic nucleus of the rat results in the excretion of a more dilute urine and
that a greater increase in plasma osmolality is needed to stimulate ADH
secretion.

Meticulous intake and output records, once- or twice-daily weight, measurement of serum electrolytes and serum and urine osmolalities, and replacement of fluid loss as free water (5% dextrose in water if given intravenously) are basic requirements of successful management. Specific drug
therapy is usually withheld in the early postoperative period until urinary
output exceeds 250 ml/hr for 2 consecutive hours or unless adequate fluid
intake cannot be maintained owing to lethargy or an impaired thirst mechanism. The rationale for this approach is that DI may be transient or progress
rapidly to the interphase of endogenous ADH secretion. However, the need
to consume large quantities of fluid may be poorly tolerated and interfere
significantly with sleep. Under these circumstances, hormone substitution
therapy may be indicated, regradless of the urinary volume.

Aqueous vasopressin (20 U/ml), because of its brief duration of action,
is the preferred agent for acute postoperative DI. The usual dose is 0.1–0.3
ml subcutaneously every 4–6 hr. The longer-acting Pitressin tannate (5 U/
ml) is the preparation most often used in the treatment of acute postoperative
DI. We have achieved good results with a starting dose of 0.25–0.5 ml
intramuscularly (1.25–2.5 U). The use of the lowest dose may result in a less
than maximally concentrated urine and its effect is dissipated more rapidly,
thus minimizing the potentially dangerous complication of water intoxication
and the less dangerous, but at times disturbing, problem of rapid shifts in
serum sodium concentration. As the effect wears off, we allow a water diuresis to persist up to several hours in anticipation of a return of endogenous
ADH secretion.

Intranasal dDAVP (2.5–5 μg) may also be used to provide an antidiuresis of up to 18 hr.[9,86] Its major disadvantage is that in unconscious patients the drug must be administered by the physician or a member of the nurs-
ing staff; this may be readily accomplished, however, by attaching one end
of the fluid-filled catheter to a syringe which is then used to expel the liquid high in the nasal cavity. Intravenous or subcutaneous dDAVP, which is
not yet available in the United States, would be more appropriate in this setting. Parenteral doses are much smaller, about one-tenth of the intranasal
dose.

REFERENCES

1. Vavra I, Machova A, Holecek V, et al: Effect of a synthetic analogue of vasopressin in animals and patients with diabetes insipidus. *Lancet* 1:948–952, 1968.
2. Andersson KE, Arner B: Effects of ddAVP, a synthetic analogue of vasopressin, in patients with cranial diabetes insipidus. *Acta Med Scand* 192:21–27, 1972.
3. Edwards CRW, Kitau MJ, Chard T, et al: Vasopressin analogue ddAVP in diabetes insipidus: Clinical and laboratory studies. *Br Med J* 3:375–378, 1973.
4. Aronson AS, Andersson KE, Bergstrand CG, et al: Treatment of diabetes insipidus in children with ddAVP, a synthetic analogue of vasopressin. *Acta Paediatr Scand* 62:133–140, 1973.
5. Kauli R, Laron Z: A vasopressin analogue in treatment of diabetes insipidus. *Arch Dis Child* 49:482–485, 1974.
6. Ward MK, Fraser TR: DDAVP in treatment of vasopressin-sensitive diabetes insipidus. *Br Med J* 3:386–389, 1974.
7. Lee W-NP, Lippe EM, LaFranchi SH, et al: Vasopressin analog DDAVP in the treatment of diabetes insipidus. *Am J Dis Child* 130:166–169, 1976.
8. Robinson AG: DDAVP in the treatment of central diabetes insipidus. *N Engl J Med* 294:507–511, 1976.
9. Cobb WE, Spare S, Reichlin S: Neurogenic diabetes insipidus: Management with ddAVP (1-desamino-8-D arginine vasopressin). *Ann Intern Med* 88:183–188, 1978.
10. Dingman JF, Hauger-Klevene JH: Treatment of diabetes insipidus: Synthetic lysine vasopressin nasal solution. *J Clin Endocrinol Metab* 24:550–553, 1964.
11. Moses AM: Synthetic lysine vasopressin nasal spray in the treatment of diabetes insipidus. *Clin Pharmacol Ther* 5:422–427, 1964.
12. Munica N, Wegienka LC, Forsham PH: Lypressin nasal spray. *J Am Med Assoc* 203:286–287, 1968.
13. Bronstein SB, DeFelice EA, Long D: Evaluation of lysine-8-vasopressin nasal spray in 641 patients with diabetes insipidus. *J Am Med Assoc* 208:1481, 1969.
14. Zaoral M, Kole J, Sorm F: Synthesis of 1-deamino-8-D-aminobutyrine vasopressin and 1-deamino-8-D-arginine vasopressin. *Coll Czech Chem Commun* 32:1250–1257, 1967.
15. Sawyer WH, Acosta M, Manning M: Structural changes in arginine vasopressin molecule that prolong its antidiuretic action. *Endocrinology* 95:140–149, 1974.
16. Sawyer WH, Acosta M, Balaspiri L, et al: Structural changes in the arginine vasopressin molecule that enhance antidiuretic activity and specificity. *Endocrinology* 94:1106–1115, 1974.
17. Seif SM, Zensen TY, Ciarochi FFF, et al: DDAVP (1-desamino-8-D-arginine-vasopressin) treatment of central diabetes insipidus—Mechanism of prolonged antidiuresis. *J Clin Endocrinol Metab* 46:381–388, 1978.
18. Jamison RL, Oliver RE: Disorders of urinary concentration and dilution. *Am J Med* 72:308–322, 1982.
19. Cort JH, Schuck O, Stribrna J, et al: Role of the disulfide bridge and the C-terminal tripeptide in the antidiuretic action of vasopressin in man and the rat. *Kidney Int* 8:292–302, 1975.
20. Dunn MJ, Kinter LB, Shier D, et al: The interactions of vasopressin and renal prostaglandins in the homozygous diabetes insipidus rat. *Clin Res* 27:496A, 1979.
21. Dunn MJ, Greely HP, Valtin H, et al: Renal excretion of prostaglandins E_2 and $F_2\alpha$ in diabetes insipidus rats. *Am J Physiol* 235:E624–627, 1978.

22. Beck TR, Hassid A, Dunn MJ: The effect of arginine vasopressin and its analogues on the synthesis of PGE$_2$ by rat renal medullary interstitial cells in culture. *J Pharm Exp Ther* 215:15–19, 1980.

23. Zusman RM: Prostaglandins, vasopressin and renal water absorption. *Med Clin N Am* 65:915–925, 1981.

24. Moses AM, Moses LK, Notman DD: Antidiuretic responses to injected desmopressin, alone and with indomethacin. *J Clin Endocrinol Metab* 52:910–913, 1981.

25. Walker RM, Brown RS, Stoff JS: Role of renal prostaglandins during antidiuresis and water diuresis in man. *Kidney Int* 21:365–370, 1982.

26. Rado JP, Marosi J, Fischer J, et al: Relationship between the dose of 1-deamino-8-D-arginine vasopressin and the antidiuretic response in man. *Endokrinologie* 66:184–185, 1975.

27. Pullan PT, Burger HG, Johnston CI: Pharmacokinetics of 1-desamino-8-D-arginine vasopressin (dDAVP) in patients with central diabetes insipidus. *Clin Endocrinol* 9:273–278, 1978.

28. Baumann G, Dingman JF: Distribution, blood transport and degradation of antidiuretic hormone in man. *J Clin Invest* 57:1109–1116, 1976.

29. Walter R, Shland H: Differences in the enzymatic inactivation of arginine vasopressin and oxytocin by rat kidney homogenate. *Endocrinology* 96:811–814, 1975.

30. Lauson HE: Metabolism of the neurohypophysial hormones, in Knobil E, Sawyer WH (eds): *Handbook of Physiology*, Section 7. Washington, DC, American Physiological Society, 1974, vol IV, pp 287–393.

31. Rado JP, Marosi J, Borbely L, et al: Individual differences in the antidiuretic response induced by DDAVP. *Horm Metab Res* 8:155–156, 1976.

32. Rado JP, Marosi J, Borbely L, et al: Individual differences in the antidiuretic response induced by single doses of 1-deamino-8-D-arginine-vasopressin (DDAVP) in patients with pituitary diabetes insipidus. *Int J Clin Pharmacol* 14:259–265, 1976.

33. Rado JP: Response to vasopressin analogues in diabetes insipidus. *N Engl J Med* 295:393, 1976.

34. Marek J, Loutocky A, Pacovsky V, et al: Ten year experience with DDAVP in treatment of diabetes insipidus. *Endokrinologie* 72:188–194, 1978.

35. Cort JH: Personal communication.

36. Oravec D, Lichardus B: Management of diabetes insipidus in pregnancy. *Br Med J* 4:114–115, 1972.

37. Burrow GN, Wassenaar W, Robertson GL, et al: DDAVP treatment of diabetes insipidus during pregnancy and the post-partum. *Acta Endocrinol* 97:23–25, 1981.

38. Hime MC, Richardson JA: Diabetes insipidus and pregnancy. Case report: Incidence and review of literature. *Obstet Gynecol Surv* 33:375–379, 1978.

39. Lampert RP, Blackett PR, Rennert OM: Management of diabetes insipidus with DDAVP. *J Pediatr* 93:896–897, 1978.

40. Robertson GL: The physiology of vasopressin (VP) excretion in man (abstract). *Clin Res* 20:778, 1972.

41. Rado JO, Marosi J, Fischer J: Shortened duration of action of 1-deamino-8-D-arginine vasopressin (DDAVP) in patients with diabetes insipidus requiring high doses of peroral antidiuretic drugs. *J Clin Pharmacol* 16:518–524, 1976.

42. Rado JP, Marosi J: Prolongation of duration of action of 1-deamino-8-argine vasopressin (DDAVP) by ineffective doses of clofibrate in diabetes insipidus. *Horm Metab Res* 7:527–528, 1975.

43. Laszlo FA, Czako L: 1-desamino-4-valine-8-D-arginine-vasopressin, a new synthetic vasopressin analog for treating diabetes insipidus. *Int J Clin Pharmacol Ther Toxicol* 20:39–43, 1982.
44. Nusynowitz ML, Forsham PH: The antidiuretic action of acetominophen. *Am J Med Sci* 252:429–435, 1966.
45. Nusynowitz ML, Wegienka LC, Bower BF, et al: Effect on vasopressin action of analgesic drugs *in vitro*. *Am J Med Sci* 252:424–428, 1966.
46. Fichman MP, Speckart P, Zia P, et al: Antidiuretic responses to prostaglandin inhibition in nephrogenic diabetes insipidus (abstract). *Clin Res* 24:161A, 1976.
47. Arduino F, Ferraz FPJ, Rodrigues J: Antidiuretic action of chlorpropamide in idiopathic diabetes insipidus. *J Clin Endocrinol Metab* 26:1325–1328, 1966.
48. Miller M, Moses AM: Mechanism of chlorpropamide action in diabetes insipidus. *J Clin Endocrinol Metab* 30:488–496, 1970.
49. Moses AM, Numann P, Miller M: Mechanism of chlorpropamide-induced antidiuresis in man: Evidence for release of ADH and enhancement of peripheral action. *Metabolism* 22:59–66, 1973.
50. Murase T, Yoshida S: Mechanism of chlorpropamide action in patients with diabetes insipidus. *J Clin Endocrinol Metab* 36:174–177, 1973.
51. Ingelfinger JR, Hayes RM: Evidence that chlorpropamide and vasopressin share a common site of action. *J Clin Endocrinol Metab* 29:738–740, 1969.
52. Beck N, Kim KS, Davis BB: Effect of chlorpropamide on cyclic AMP in rat renal medulla. *Endocrinology* 95:771–774, 1974.
53. Mendoza S: Effect of chlorpropamide on the permeability of urinary bladder of the toad and the response to vasopressin, adenosine 3′,5′-monophosphate and theophylline. *Endocrinology* 84:411–416, 1969.
54. Miller M, Moses AM: Potentiation of vasopressin action by chlorpropamide *in vivo*. *Endocrinology* 86:1024, 1970.
55. Moses AM, Coulson R: Augmentation by chlorpropamide of 1-deamino-8-D-arginine vasopressin-induced antidiuresis and stimulation of renal medullary adenylate cyclase and accumulation of adenosine 3′5′-monophosphate. *Endocrinology* 106:967–974, 1980.
56. Moses AM, Fenner R, Schroeder ET, et al: Further studies on the mechanism by which chlorpropamide alters the action of vasopressin. *Endocrinology* 111:2025–2030, 1982.
57. Zusman RM, Keiser HR, Handler JS: Inhibition of vasopressin-stimulated prostaglandin E biosynthesis by chlorpropamide in the toad urinary bladder: Mechanism of enhancement of vasopressin-stimulated water flow. *J Clin Invest* 60:1348–1353, 1977.
58. Pokracki FJ, Robinson AG, Seif SM: Chlorpropamide effect: Measure of neurophysin and vasopressin in humans and rats. *Metabolism* 30:72–78, 1981.
59. Webster B, Bain J: Antidiuretic effect and complications of chlorpropamide therapy in diabetes insipidus. *J Clin Endocrinol Metab* 30:215–217, 1970.
60. Wales JK, Fraser TR: The clinical use of chlorpropamide in diabetes insipidus. *Acta Endocrinol* 68:725–736, 1971.
61. Fichman MP, Vorherr H, Kleeman CR, et al: Diuretic-induced hyponatremia. *Ann Intern Med* 75:853–863, 1971.
62. Rado JP: Combination of carbamazepine and chlorpropamide in the treatment of "hyporesponder" pituitary diabetes insipidus. *J Clin Endocrinol* 38:1–7, 1974.
63. Mahoney JH, Goodman AD: Hypernatremia due to hypodipsia and elevated threshold for vasopressin release: Effects of treatment with hydrochlorothiazide, chlorpropamide and tolbutamide. *N Engl J Med* 279:1191, 1968.

162   WILLIAM E. COBB

64. Bode HN, Harey DM, Crawford JD: Restoration of normal drinking behavior by chlorpro-
    pamide in patients with hypodipsia and diabetes insipidus. Am J Med 51:304–309, 1971.
65. Plum F, Titert RV: Nonendocrine diseases and disorders of the hypothalamus, in Reichlin
    S, Baldessarini RJ, Martin JB (eds): The Hypothalamus. New York, Raven Press, 1978,
    pp 415–473.
66. Moses AM, Howanitz J, van Gemert M, et al: Clofibrate-induced antidiuresis. J Clin Invest
    52:535–542, 1973.
67. Bonnici F: Antidiuretic effects of clofibrate and carbamazepine in diabetes insipidus: Studies
    on free water clearance and response to a water load. Clin Endocrinol 2:265–275, 1973.
68. Thompson P: Comparison of clofibrate and chlorpropamide in vasopressin-responsive dia-
    betes insipidus. Metabolism 26:749–762, 1977.
69. Kimura T, Matsui K, Sato T, et al: Mechanism of carbamazepine (Tegretol)-induced an-
    tidiuresis: Evidence for release of antidiuretic hormone and impaired excretion of water
    load. J Clin Endocrinol Metab 38:356–362, 1974.
70. Meindes AE, Cejka V, Robertson GL: The antidiuretic action of carbamazepine in man.
    Clin Soc Mol Med 47:289–299, 1974.
71. Wales JK: Treatment of diabetes insipidus with carbamazepine. Lancet 2:948–951, 1975.
72. Crawford JD, Kennedy GC: Animal physiology: Chlorothiazide in diabetes insipidus. Nature
    183:891–892, 1959.
73. Kuman RT, Weller DR, Webb HL: Clarification of the site of action of chlorothiazide in
    the rat nephron. J Clin Invest 56:401–407, 1975.
74. Earley LE, Arloff J: The mechanism of antidiuresis associated with the administration of
    hydrochlorothiazide to patients with vasopressin-resistant diabetes insipidus. J Clin Invest
    41:1988–1997, 1962.
75. Randall RV, Clark EC, Dodge HW Jr, et al: Polyuria after operations for tumors in the
    region of the hypophysis and hypothalamus. J Clin Endocrinol Metab 20:1614–1621, 1960.
76. Sharkey PC, Perry JG, Ehni G: Diabetes insipidus following section of hypophyseal stalk.
    J Neurosurg 18:445–460, 1961.
77. Fisher C, Ingram WR, Ranson SW: Diabetes insipidus and the neurohormonal control of
    water balance: A contribution to the structure and function of the hypothalamo-hypophysial
    system. Ann Arbor, MI, Edwards Brothers, 1938.
78. Laszlo FA, de Wied D: Antidiuretic hormone content of the hypothalamo-neurohypophysial
    system and urinary excretion of antidiuretic hormone in rats during the development of
    diabetes insipidus after lesions in the pituitary stalk. J Endocrinol 36:125–137, 1966.
79. Kovacs K, Laszlo FA, David MA: The antidiuretic phase of water metabolism in rats after
    lesions of the pituitary stalk. II. The role of the antidiuretic hormone. J Endocrinol 25:397–401,
    1962.
80. Shucart WA, Jackson I: Management of diabetes insipidus in neurosurgical patients. J
    Neurosurg 44:65–71, 1976.
81. Cobb WE: Endocrine management after pituitary surgery, in Post KD, Jackson IMD, Reichlin
    S (eds): The Pituitary Adenoma. New York, Plenum Medical, 1980, pp 417–435.
82. Wen-hsien W, Zbuzek VK: Vasopressin and anesthesia surgery. Bull NY Acad Sci 58:427–442,
    1982.
83. Moses AM, Miller J, Streeten DHP: Pathophysiologic and pharmacologic alterations in the
    release and action of ADH. Metabolism 25:697–721, 1976.
84. Aubry RH, Nankin HR, Moses AM, et al: Measurement of the osmotic threshold for
    vasopressin release in human subjects, and its modification by cortisol. J Clin Endocrinol
    Metab 25:1481–1492, 1965.

85. Streeten DHP, Ross GS, Souma M: Osmotic threshold for ADH release: Effects of cortisol introduced into supra-optic nuclei. Presented at the 5th Meeting of the Endocrine Society, Chicago, June 20–22, 1973.
86. Daneman DD, Ehrlich RM, Bailey JD: Postcraniotomy diabetes insipidus: Treatment with DDAVP, a synthetic analog of vasopressin. *J Pediatr* 93:879–880, 1978.

9

SYNDROME OF INAPPROPRIATE ANTIDIURETIC HORMONE SECRETION

Susan Hou

1. INTRODUCTION

In 1957, Schwartz, Bennett, Curelop, and Bartter described two patients with bronchogenic carcinoma who had developed hyponatremia despite continued urinary sodium loss.[1] They noted that the syndrome was similar to the response of normal individuals given an infusion of pitressin and water, and they postulated that the tumor led to inappropriate release of antidiuretic hormone (ADH).

In their original study and in a second paper ten years later,[2] Schwartz and his colleagues discussed the cardinal features of the entity that has come to be known as the syndrome of inappropriate antidiuretic hormone secretion (SIADH). These include (1) hyponatremia with hypoosmolality of serum and extracellular fluid, (2) continued renal excretion of sodium, (3) absence of clinical evidence of volume depletion or edema, (4) inappropriately high urine osmolality, (5) normal renal function, and (6) normal adrenal function.

Susan Hou • Department of Internal Medicine, St. Margaret's Hospital for Women, Boston, Massachusetts 02125; and Department of Medicine, Tufts University School of Medicine, Boston, Massachusetts 02111.

2. THE CLINICAL PROBLEMS IN PATIENTS WITH SIADH

In reviewing the consequences of chronic hyponatremia Arieff and Guisado have noted thirst, impaired taste, and anorexia accompanied by dyspnea on exertion, fatigue, and dulled sensorium when the serum sodium falls rapidly from 147 to 131 mEq/liter. More severe gastrointestinal symptoms such as nausea, vomiting, and abdominal cramps occur if the sodium drops to 120–130 mEq/liter.[3]

When the serum sodium falls below 115 mEq/liter, confusion, lethargy, muscle twitching, and convulsions may occur.

ADH normally leads to water reabsorption in the collecting duct. If present in excess, ADH-induced water retention leads to dilutional hyponatremia. Volume expansion resulting from water retention leads to an increase in glomerular filtration rate and increased clearance of urea and creatinine. Concentrations in blood of these substances are frequently at the lower end of normal [blood urea nitrogen (BUN) less than 10 mg/dl, creatinine between 0.4 and 0.7 mg/dl]. Hypouricemia is the rule in patients with SIADH. Beck found the mean serum uric acid concentration in 17 patients with SIADH to be 2.9 mg/dl (highest value slightly over 4 mg/dl), in contrast to a mean value of 7.7 mg/dl in patients with other causes of hyponatremia.[4]

Sodium reabsorption in the proximal tubule is determined by intravascular volume rather than serum sodium concentration, although the nature of the signal to the proximal tubule, the so-called third factor, remains to be identified.[5] In the presence of volume expansion, proximal tubular sodium reabsorption is suppressed and urine sodium is high.

Patients with SIADH usually retain 2–5 liters of excess water. Schwartz et al. noted that most patients with SIADH reached a new steady state with serum sodiums ranging from slightly below normal to 100–110 mEq/liter. When the new steady state is reached, patients are no longer in negative sodium balance and sodium excretion matches intake. In SIADH induced experimentally by prolonged infusion of Pitressin®, sodium excretion and urine osmolality fall toward control values in 7–10 days. Schwartz et al. suggested several explanations for the achievement of a new steady state. These include an increase in proximal tubular pressure and luminal radius, a reduction of medullary hypertonicity, resulting in decreased water reabsorption in the loop of Henle, and a decrease in permeability of the distal nephron to water.[2]

Because the water retained in SIADH is distributed into total body water, only 25% goes into the interstitial spaces and the patients do not appear edematous; weight gain can be detected if they are observed while hyponatremia is developing. In the presence of hyponatremia one expects the urine to be maximally dilute; inappropriately high urine osmolality is a hallmark of the syndrome.

SIADH is generally associated with nearly normal serum potassium and bicarbonate levels. Several factors determine potassium excretion. As the syndrome develops, aldosterone secretion and thus potassium secretion are first suppressed by volume expansion, while increased delivery of sodium to the distal tubule increases potassium excretion by increasing luminal negativity[5] and less importantly by increasing carrier-mediated potassium flow. The increased flow through the distal tubule increases potassium excretion because equilibration is rapid and the volume of tubular fluid limits the rate of potassium excretion. However, severe serum hypotonicity leads to increased aldosterone secretion; at levels of serum sodium below 115 mEq/liter, aldosterone secretion occurs despite volume expansion. Elevated aldosterone levels result in increased potassium secretion in the distal tubule. In individuals with SIADH, increased aldosterone secretion prevents bicarbonate loss despite depressed proximal reabsorption of the sodium, which would usually be accompanied by bicarbonate loss. The effects of aldosterone on bicarbonate conservation have been demonstrated in dogs made acidotic with HCl infusions.[6] Brain cells are protected from the effects of hyperosmolar states by newly formed cerebral osmotically active substances referred to as idiogenic osmoles.[7] The converse is true in SIADH. Schwartz et al. noted that the degree of hypoosmolality is not accounted for by water retention and sodium loss. They postulated that inactivation of intracellular osmoles may occur slowly and explain the greater tolerance of the brain to slowly developing hyponatremia than to rapidly developing hyponatremia.

The development of a reliable assay for ADH confirmed the hypothesis of Schwartz and his colleagues that in the syndrome they had described ADH levels are inappropriately high in relation to serum tonicity. In some cases, levels are higher than are ever produced under normal circumstances. After the development of ADH assays, Robertson and his colleagues described four patterns of ADH release seen in 47 patients with the hyponatremia of SIADH.[8]

In Robertson's Type A (20% of patients), there are wide swings in ADH levels and ADH secretion shows no evidence of control by osmotic stimuli.

In Type B SIADH (35% of patients), ADH levels rise in response to hypertonic saline infusion and the ADH rise parallels the normal curve. However, ADH secretion is fully suppressed only at a very low serum osmolality. DeFronzo and his colleagues[9] also described four patients with this pattern. These patients had chronic hyponatremia with serum sodium levels of between 125 and 132 mEq/liter. All were able to dilute their urine to less than 100 mOsm/kg. When given a high-sodium diet, they remained in sodium balance without correcting their hyponatremia. Three corrected their hyponatremia after treatment of their underlying problem, which was pulmonary tuberculosis in two cases.[9]

In Type C (35% of patients), plasma ADH levels increase appropriately during hypertonic saline infusion, but ADH release cannot be completely suppressed regardless of the severity of the hypotonicity. This pattern of continuous, nonsuppressible ADH production was noted in several patients with neurologic disease.

In Type D (10% of patients), ADH secretion is entirely normal but the urine remains inappropriately concentrated, suggesting either a change in renal sensitivity to ADH or a different, as yet unidentified, antidiuretic substance.

3. CAUSES OF SIADH (Table I)

3.1. Cancer

The original report of SIADH included two patients with bronchogenic carcinoma.[1] The mechanism by which the tumor produced increased ADH was not known. Hypotheses included production of ADH by the tumor, stimulation of intrathoracic volume receptors by the tumor, or production of a substance that stimulates pituitary ADH release. In 1963, Amatruda and his colleagues reported a patient with bronchogenic carcinoma in whom bioassay identified ADH in extracts of the tumor.[10] Bower and his colleagues[11] reported a patient with SIADH and oat cell carcinoma of the lung in whom ADH activity was markedly elevated in a hepatic metastasis but not in the irradiated primary tumor. SIADH was present despite destruction of the posterior pituitary by metastasis.[11] Radioimmunoassay substantiates the ADH-like nature of the bioactive substance found in these patients.[12] Early in the historic development of the concept of ectopic hormone secretion by tumors, the suggestion was made that circulating ADH was taken up by tumors rather

TABLE I. Causes of SIADH

Cancer	Neurologic (*cont.*)
Oat cell carcinoma of the lung	Porphyria (acute intermittent)
Adenocarcinoma of the lung	Subarachnoid bleeding
Carcinoma of the duodenum	Cerebrovascular thrombosis
Carcinoma of the pancreas	Lung
Thymoma	Pneumonia
Squamous cell carcinoma of the tongue	Tuberculosis
Leukemia	Aspergillosis
Hodgkin's disease	Postoperative
Lymphoma	Psychiatric disease
Neurologic	Drugs (see Table II)
Meningitis	Miscellaneous
Head injuries	Myocardial infarction
Brain tumor	Malaria
Brain abscess	Measles
Encephalitis	Idiopathic
Guillain–Barré syndrome	

than produced by them. Yamaji and his colleagues[13] found immunoreactive ADH with molecular weights of 10,000–20,000 in oat cell carcinoma. When the tissue was incubated with radiolabeled cysteine, the labeled amino acid appeared first in the 20,000-molecular-weight neurophysins. Incubation of 20,000-molecular-weight neurophysin with trypsin yielded equimolar amounts of the 10,000-molecular-weight neurophysin and of ADH. These findings suggest that the 20,000-molecular-weight neurophysin is the precursor to both ADH and the smaller neurophysin. Incorporation of a radiolabeled amino acid precursor is evidence that synthesis of ADH and neurophysin has taken place in the tumor.

Odell and his colleagues have suggested that, although clinically important syndromes associated with ectopic hormone secretion are rare, production of peptide hormones by tumors is extremely common.[14] They measured the concentrations of vasopressin and vasotocin (an analogue normally found only in lower animal forms) in an assay that measured both peptides in the blood of patients with 64 tumors who had no clinical evidence of ectopic hormone production. Vasopressin and vasotocin were identified in 41% of patients with lung cancers and 43% of patients with colon cancer. Extracts of tumor tissue contained higher concentrations of vasopressin and vasotocin than did normal tissues.[14] In 14 patients with lung cancer without clinical SIADH, Padfield et al. found that plasma ADH levels were higher than in normals.[12] These studies suggest that secretion of peptide hormone is common in neoplasms, particularly in oat cell carcinomas of the lung. Odell et al.[14] noted no response to regulatory stimuli while Padfield et al. showed an ADH response to fluid restriction suggestive of some degree of physiologic control. Therefore, these patients may fall into both Robertson's categories A and B.

Other tumors that have been reported in association with SIADH are listed in Table I.

3.2. Neurohypophysial Trauma

Following damage by trauma or surgery to the supraoptic and paraventricular nuclei of the hypothalamus or high pituitary stalk disruption, a triphasic pattern of ADH release ensues in most patients. The experimental model was first described by Fisher et al. in 1938.[15] The first phase is characterized by diabetes insipidus owing to acute interference with ADH secretion, a phase lasting 1–7 days. The second phase is a period of inappropriate ADH secretion as stored ADH is released in an unregulated fashion from axon terminals in the posterior pituitary. If stalk section is 90–100% complete, the latent phase when ADH is secreted is followed by permanent diabetes insipidus.

Transient SIADH frequently occurs following pituitary surgery even in the absence of any permanent damage to the hypothalamo-neurohypophysial unit. In rare instances, SIADH persists for months or years.[16]

3.3. Neurologic Disease

SIADH has been described in a wide variety of neurologic diseases. Kaplan and Feigin reported evidence of SIADH in 50% of children with bacterial meningitis. They also noted that the presence and duration of SIADH in these children had prognostic value, in that hyponatremia of long duration was associated with neurologic abnormalities at one- and three-month follow-up and with delayed development at one year. Kaplan and Feigin measured serum ADH levels in 13 normal children, 21 children hospitalized with a febrile illness (including 3 hospitalized with encephalitis and 3 with pneumonia), and 17 children hospitalized with bacterial meningitis.[17] Children with meningitis had significantly higher vasopressin levels than the other two groups. When ADH levels were studied in relationship to serum sodium, the differences become more marked. High levels of ADH persisted in the face of hyponatremia. Two children had levels that were in the "normal range" but were inappropriately high in view of their hyponatremia. Ten children had markedly increased ADH levels but were not hyponatremic.

SIADH was noted in 12 of 854 infants admitted to a neonatal intensive care unit, 11 of whom were premature.[18] SIADH began between 5 and 16 days after birth. The lowest serum sodium in these children was 116 mEq/ liter. All of the babies who developed SIADH had had serious neurologic insults during their course, including birth asphyxia, intracranial hemorrhage, or meningitis. Nine of the premature infants have been followed for long periods; seven of the nine had severe neurologic sequelae and only four had normal intelligence. These data suggest that SIADH is indicative of a severe degree of neurologic damage. In neurologic disease it appears that ADH production cannot be suppressed, even in the presence of severe hyponatremia. Therefore, such patients would fall into Robertson's Type C.

The hyponatremia seen in patients following neurosurgery has been attributed to SIADH.[19] These patients resemble those with SIADH in that they are hyponatremic and have high urinary sodium, an inappropriately high urine osmolality without clinical volume contraction or renal or adrenal dysfunction. However, the accepted pathogenesis of the hyponatremia in postoperative neurosurgical patients has been called into question by Nelson and his colleagues, who measured blood volume in 12 postoperative neurosurgical patients and found it to be decreased. They postulated that hyponatremia was caused by intravascular volume contraction and ADH release in response to volume change.[20]

SIADH has been noted in many other neurologic diseases. Joynt et al. found ADH levels to be significantly elevated in 17 patients with cerebral infarction and 4 with subarachnoid bleeding when compared to healthy controls.[21] However, the patients he studied did not have hyponatremia. He attributes the infrequency of hyponatremia to careful monitoring of electrolytes and restriction of free water and notes that there are case reports of hyponatremia in patients with strokes.[21]

Ludwig and Goldberg found hyponatremia in eight patients during attacks of acute intermittent porphyria.[22] All patients had severe neurologic involvement in the attacks of porphyria, and the underlying neurologic picture was confused by hyponatremia.

3.4. Postoperative SIADH

Following surgery of any kind, secretion of ADH is increased. The increase begins in the first few postoperative hours and persists for 5–7 days.[23] This results in only mild hyponatremia unless excessive quantities of hypotonic fluid are administered. In elderly patients, the increased ADH secretion may be more prolonged and the SIADH may become apparent as late as the tenth postoperative day.[24]

A number of factors contribute to the intraoperative and postoperative ADH release. Anesthesia lowers the threshold for ADH release in volume contraction by blocking the sympathetic reflexes that ordinarily compensate for mild volume contraction. Anesthesia also appears to increase urine osmolality in the absence of volume contraction. In many patients, the rise can be blocked by ethanol administration, suggesting that it is mediated by ADH release rather than by decreased glomerular filtration rate or decreased renal plasma flow.[2]

Intubation and positive-pressure breathing either during or after surgery result in ADH release secondary to decreased intrathoracic blood flow. Left atrial receptors respond to decreased intrathoracic blood flow as they would to volume contraction.[25] Postoperative pain is associated with increased ADH secretion.[26] The effect of narcotics on ADH release in humans is a subject of controversy. Philbin et al. found no rise in ADH levels mesured by radioimmunoassay during morphine anesthesia. However, ADH levels increased with surgical manipulations, and they attribute previously reported ADH-like activity in patients receiving morphine to factors such as pain, effect on left atrial volume receptors, and surgical manipulation.[27] The administration of β-endorphin results in an increase in plasma ADH levels, suggesting that the ADH response to pain may be mediated by endorphins.[28]

3.5. SIADH Associated with Pulmonary Disease

SIADH has been described in a number of infectious pulmonary diseases, most commonly tuberculosis, but also including bacterial,[29] viral,[30] and mycoplasma pneumonia.[31] One hypothesis advanced to explain the development of hyponatremia in the setting of severe pneumonia is that it causes decreased pulmonary perfusion secondary to the pulmonary vasoconstriction associated with hypoxia. Moreover, the areas of pneumonia in the lung appear as avascular segments on perfusion studies. These two changes may lead to a decrease in the pressure perceived by left atrial volume receptors. These receptors decrease vagal afferent activity and increase activity of the neurohypophysis.

Another explanation that has been advanced is that infected lung tissue produces ADH. A single report by Vorherr and his colleagues describes the finding of bioassayable ADH in tuberculous lung tissue in a patient with hyponatremia.[32]

The greater frequency of SIADH in pulmonary infections compared to other types of infection and the wide range of organisms involved make changes in pulmonary perfusion the more plausible explanation.

3.6. SIADH Associated with Endocrine Disorders

In the original description of SIADH, normal adrenal function was one of the criteria required to make the diagnosis. However, ADH plays a role in the hyponatremia associated with adrenal, thyroid, and anterior pituitary insufficiency; these disorders may be regarded as special forms of SIADH.

Many studies have shown that myxedema is frequently accompanied by hyponatremia and that, with no therapy other than replacement of thyroid hormone, water excretion returns to normal. The impairment of renal water excretion was initially attributed to changes in renal plasma flow, leading to proximal tubular sodium avidity and decreased delivery of filtrate to the diluting segments of the distal tubule.[33]

Subsequent investigators have postulated that inappropriately elevated ADH levels may have contributed to the hyponatremia in myxedema. Skowsky and Kikuchi measured the plasma vasopressin levels in 20 myxedematous patients given a standard water load before and after treatment of their hypothyroidism.[34] The myxedematous patients excreted a mean of 49.4% of the water load at 4 hr. Plasma osmolality dropped to a mean of 268.6 mOsm/kg and urine osmolality was not suppressed normally, the mean urine osmolality being 169.8 mOsm/kg. Osmolar clearance was the same for hypothyroid and euthyroid patients. Eight patients were studied after treatment of their hypothyroidism, and water excretion had returned to normal, the mean percentage of water excreted by 4 hr rising to 93.4%. The cardiac index was normal prior to thyroid hormone replacement, making increased sodium avidity secondary to decreased blood volume in myxedema unlikely. Basal ADH levels were abnormally high in 14 of the 20 patients. Of the hypothyroid patients only five showed normal suppression of ADH with a water load. Of these five only two had normal urinary dilution, suggesting a primary renal diluting defect in the other three.

From the study of myxedematous patients with normal excretion of a water load and minimum urine osmolalities only slightly higher than when they become euthyroid, other investigators have concluded that a reset osmostat is the mechanism by which the patients develop hyponatremia.[35] A patient with myxedema has been described in whom ADH appeared to play no role in causing hyponatremia.[36] Urine osmolality did not fall following administration of demeclocycline (see Section 5.2), and ADH levels were appropriately suppressed.[36] Therefore, a number of mechanisms have been proposed to explain the hyponatremia found in myxedema, and it is possible that this condition may have different etiologies in individual patients or that in a single patient more than one mechanism may be operative.

ADH appears to play a role in the water excreting defect in adrenal cortical and in anterior pituitary insufficiency. Agus and Goldberg studied water excretion in seven patients with anterior pituitary insufficiency, one of whom had adrenal deficiency as well.[37] In the group with anterior pituitary insufficiency given thyroid hormone replacement, four patients could not dilute their urine in response to a water load (Group I) and three diluted their urine in response to a water load; however, the dilution was transient and they began concentrating their urine again after a short time. The administration of hydrocortisone improved urinary dilution in both groups. The effect was dose-related, Group I patients requiring higher doses. Ethanol caused no change in urinary osmolality in Group I patients, but in Group II patients it made the urine remain hypotonic if given before the increase in osmolality. Submaximal doses of hydrocortisone converted the response of Group I to a pattern similar to that of Group II. When hydrocortisone was given to patients with posterior hypopituitarism and diabetes insipidus during constant vasopressin administration, it had no effect. The findings of Agus and Goldberg indicate that while hydrocortisone is necessary for normal urinary dilution, it acts by modulating ADH release. In patients with diabetes insipidus undergoing a vasopressin infusion, the administration of hydrocortisone causes no change in urinary dilution. The change in response to ethanol with the administration of hydrocortisone suggests that hydrocortisone is necessary for a posterior pituitary response to common stimuli. Further evidence of the role of ADH in the hyponatremia associated with adrenal deficiency is seen in the response of mineralocorticoid- and glucocorticoid-deficient rats given an ADH antagonist (1-β-mercapto-β,β-cyclopenta-methylenepropionic acid 2-O-ethyltyrosine, 4-valine AVP). Administration of the compound improves the ability of both mineralocorticoid- and glucocorticoid-deficient rats to excrete a water load and decreases their minimum urine osmolality.[38]

3.7. Psychiatric Disorders

Hyponatremia caused by compulsive water ingestion is sometimes difficult to differentiate from SIADH caused by psychiatric disease. Cases of hyponatremia caused by uncomplicated psychogenic polydipsia have been reported. Linshaw et al. describe three infants with psychogenic polydipsia, one of whom had a serum sodium of 132 mOsm/kg and urine specific gravity of 1.002.[39] Many other children with uncomplicated psychogenic polydipsia without neurologic or renal disease have had normal serum sodiums.[40] Hyponatremia is more common when SIADH associated with psychiatric disease is accompanied by psychogenic polydipsia. Hariprasad and his colleagues described 20 psychotic patients with combined psychogenic polydipsia and a urinary diluting defect suggestive of SIADH on the basis of reset osmostat, compatible with Robertson's Type B.[41] In these patients serum sodium ranged from 98 to 124 mEq/liter. During self-induced water loading in seven of these patients, urine osmolality ranged from 37 to 102 mOsm/kg with a value of under 100 mOsm/kg in six of seven patients, indicating that they were able to dilute their urine maximally. During fluid restriction, these patients began to concentrate their urine while plasma osmolality was still decreased. The explanation suggested by these authors for the inappropriately high urine concentration is that the "osmostat" is reset so that urine can be diluted maximally, but only when the patient has become severely hypoosmotic; in addition there is a change in responsiveness of volume receptors. An important associated change in psychogenic polydipsia is marked hypokalemia. Increased flow through the distal tubule increases the potassium excretion. Urine sodium concentration in patients of Hariprasad[41] ranged from 0 to 6 mEq/liter, but sodium excretion would be expected to equal sodium intake when they reached a steady state. Since fluid intake ranged from 7 to 43 liters (with production of maximally dilute urine some 28 liters may be excreted), this high volume led to excretion of a substantial amount of ingested sodium. Drugs used in the treatment of psychosis are among those which cause SIADH (see Section 3.9); of the patients in this study,[33] three had not been on medication for several years.

Dubovsky et al. described one woman who developed polydipsia with

inappropriately concentrated urine during two exacerbations of schizophre-
nia.[42] Her polydipsia and altered concentrating ability resolved with improvement in her psychiatric disease.

3.8. Idiopathic SIADH

SIADH may appear transiently and resolve without a cause having been
identified. Idiopathic SIADH that persists without apparent cause is extremely
rare. Epstein et al. followed a patient with SIADH for 28 years who never
demonstrated endocrine or neurologic abnormalities.[43] She continued to manifest hyponatremia when her daily water intake exceeded 200 ml until she
was treated with demeclocycline. Whitaker et al. describe a 15-year-old patient
with SIADH and inability to maximally dilute her urine.[44] She had excessive
thirst and hypertension as well as high ADH levels. In this patient, low
intelligence and hyperactivity suggest a neurologic problem, but the neurologic damage may have been due to her long standing hyponatremia. A child
who developed hyponatremia at 3 months of age and who had intermittent
SIADH was reported by Skowsky and Fisher.[45] She was followed for almost
4 years and no tumor or CNS cause of SIADH was identified.[45] There are
two other reported cases of idiopathic SIADH, one with episodic secretion
and one with sustained secretion.[46,47]

3.9. Drug-Induced SIADH

Hyponatremia with a clinical picture identical to SIADH has been described after treatment with a variety of drugs (Table II).

3.9.1. Hypoglycemic Agents

Of patients taking chlorpropamide, 4% will develop hyponatremia while
maintaining an ordinary water intake; water loading will induce hyponatremia
in an even larger proportion of patients.[48] Chlorpropamide influences water
excretion in two ways. It appears to increase the action of circulating ADH
on the collecting duct and to stimulate ADH release. The drug has no effect
in homozygous Brattleboro rats, who have complete ADH deficiency, but it

TABLE II. Drugs Causing Hyponatremia

Hypoglycemic agents	Antipsychotic medications (*cont.*)
Chlorpropamide	Haloperidol
Tolbutamide	Diuretics
Antineoplastic agents	Hydrochlorothiazide
Cytoxan	Metolazone
Vincristine	Furosemide
Antipsychotic medications	Miscellaneous
Tranylcypromine sulfate	Clofibrate
Fluphenazine	Synthetic hormones
Thioridazine	ADH
Amitryptaline	Oxytocin

increases the effectiveness of infused ADH in these animals. It is ineffective when used in patients with diabetes insipidus with low levels of circulating ADH, although hyponatremia has been described in one such patient following chlorpropamide overdose. Chlorpropamide also appears to increase secretion of ADH. In normal individuals, the effect of chlorpropamide has been variable, but the induction of a water excretory defect in at least half of normal overhydrated individuals suggests that chlorpropamide induces ADH release since ADH is not secreted by such individuals under normal circumstances. Normal subjects treated with chlorpropamide showed an increase in urinary ADH. Since chlorpropamide does not change the metabolism of exogenous ADH, the increase in urinary ADH must be a result of increased release.[49]

The mechanism by which chlorpropamide increases ADH-mediated water flow has been studied in toad bladder.[50] In this tissue, ADH action leads to increased cyclic AMP (cAMP) production, and both ADH and cAMP increase water flow. In the presence of ADH, prostaglandin E (PGE) is produced at an increased rate and in turn limits ADH-mediated water flow. Chlorpropamide decreases the production of PGE and thereby prolongs the effect of ADH. When PGE synthesis is blocked by Naprosyn®, the effect of chlorpropamide is to decrease water flow.

The effect of chlorpropamide on water retention may become clinically evident in patients with diabetes mellitus treated with the drug because it adds to preexisting abnormalities of water metabolism. Well controlled diabetic subjects have slightly elevated plasma ADH levels and poorly controlled diabetics have markedly increased ADH. The effects of ADH are usually obscured by the osmotic diuresis caused by hyperglycemia, but water retention may occur when chlorpropamide is used to treat the hyperglycemia.[51]

A water excreting defect has been seen rarely with the use of tolbutamide, but it cannot be induced in normal individuals when the drug is taken in doses in the range used to treat diabetes mellitus.[52] SIADH has not been observed with acetohexamide or tolazamide, two other agents used for blood sugar control.

3.9.2. Antineoplastic Agents

Several drugs used in the treatment of neoplasia have been noted to cause SIADH. DeFronzo and his colleagues reported the development of a water excretory defect in 17 of 19 patients treated with parenteral cyclophospha-mide.[53] These patients had normal water loading tests when not being treated with cyclophosphamide. Four to eight hours after receiving cyclophosphamide they had a rise in urine osmolality, weight gain averaging 2 kg, drop in serum sodium of 3–20 mEq/liter, fall in serum osmolality, and persisting urinary sodium excretion. The patient groups included ten patients with leukemia, a disorder that has only rarely been associated with SIADH,[54] and one patient with aplastic anemia. The time course of the water excreting defect paralleled urinary excretion of an active metabolite of cyclophosphamide, and the water excretory defect resolved in 20 hr or less. Cyclophosphamide-induced SIADH is clinically important because patients treated with this drug are usually hydrated vigorously to protect against hemorrhagic cystitis.

Severe hyponatremia has been reported to follow treatment with vincristine. A report of a single patient by Cutting describes the development of severe hyponatremia accompanied by weight gain and continued excretion of sodium on the eighth day after high-dose vincristine administration.[55] The hypothesis has been advanced that inappropriate release of ADH occurs because of neurotoxic effects of vincristine affecting the posterior pituitary.

3.9.3. Neuroleptics and Other Neuroactive Agents

A water excretory defect similar to SIADH has been reported with the use of carbamazepine (Tegretol®), amitriptyline, thioridazine (Mellaril®),[52] and the monoamine oxidase inhibitor tranylcypromine sulfate.[56] These drugs probably act centrally to increase ADH release. Carbamazepine has been demonstrated to increase ADH release and has no effect on ADH action. In patients with partial diabetes insipidus, carbamazepine increases serum ADH levels. This effect can be blocked by ethanol administration. It has no effect in Brattleboro rats, who have complete ADH deficiency, and it has no direct action on the toad bladder. The water excretory defect caused by these drugs has become evident when they are used in patients with a high water intake.

3.9.4. Clofibrate

Clofibrate, a cholesterol-lowering drug, has been used in the treatment of partial diabetes insipidus, in preference to chlorpropamide because it does not carry the risk of hypoglycemia. It works by increasing ADH release from the posterior pituitary. It does not increase the action of exogenously administered ADH.[57] Clofibrate gives rise to an abnormal water loading test in normal volunteers but does not produce clinically important hyponatremia.

3.9.5. Diuretics

Fichman and his colleagues described 25 patients who developed severe hyponatremia while taking thiazide diuretics, furosemide or chlorthalidone.[58] All appeared euvolemic on physical examination. The serum sodium levels in this group of patients ranged from 91 to 120 mEq/liter; hyponatremia disappeared 3–10 days after stopping diuretics and reappeared within 2–12 days after rechallenge. Although the group did not appear to be volume-contracted, the highest serum creatinine values in the group (up to 1.2 mg%) were normal but were somewhat higher than is usual in SIADH. Bioassay showed 1–15 U ADH/ml of plasma, in contrast to the finding that levels of ADH in control subjects are unmeasurable. These workers noted that in their 22 patients the serum potassium was 3.5 mEq/liter or below and that serum bicarbonate ranged from 25 to 40 mEq/liter. The authors postulated that hypokalemia caused transport of sodium into cells, leading to a decrease in intravascular volume, which in turn resulted in ADH release mediated by volume receptors. The hyponatremia was corrected with potassium replacement. Ashraf and his colleagues have challenged the hypothesis of Fichman et al., noting that in one of Ashraf's seven patients the serum potassium was normal when hyponatremia developed during rechallenge with the drug.[59] The role of ADH in diuretic-induced hyponatremia remains controversial while these drugs remain an important cause of hyponatremia.

The consequence of diuretic-induced hyponatremia can be catastrophic.

Ashraf and his colleagues reported seven cases of thiazide-induced hyponatremia, of whom two died and two were left with severe permanent neurologic impairment.[59]

To date no drugs have been noted to have an intrinsic ADH-like action. All work either by stimulating ADH release or by potentiating circulating ADH.

4. DIFFERENTIAL DIAGNOSIS

SIADH must be distinguished from other causes of hyponatremia, which include edema-forming states, severe volume contraction, and renal insufficiency. The cause of SIADH should be determined as early as possible.

A careful history of drug ingestion, symptoms of endocrine disorders, hepatic cirrhosis, congestive heart failure, or history of volume losses is helpful, as is a history of neoplastic, neurologic, or pulmonary diseases associated with the syndrome.

On physical examination, patients with SIADH appear euvolemic. That is, they do not appear edematous, hypertensive, or plethoric. Edema, if present, suggests that congestive heart failure, cirrhosis, or nephrotic syndrome is responsible for the hyponatremia. Patients with volume contraction severe enough to cause hyponatremia usually have decreased skin turgor and postural hypotension. Patients with SIADH secondary to hypothyroidism are usually severely myxedematous. The mean T4 in Skowsky's patients was 1.4 mg/dl. Such patients usually but not invariably have typical changes of hypothyroidism on examination. Patients with adrenal cortical deficiency are often volume-contracted and often have postural hypotension but many appear euvolemic, and often the diagnosis cannot be made on physical examination.

Several laboratory determinations are helpful. The cardinal laboratory finding is serum hyponatremia and hypoosmolality unaccompanied by laboratory findings of volume contraction, which include elevation of serum BUN, creatinine, and uric acid. Urine sodium is helpful in distinguishing SIADH from other conditions that cause hyponatremia. Urine sodium is low in congestive heart failure, cirrhosis, nephrotic syndrome, and volume contraction owing to electrolyte loss. Although ADH may play some role in the hyponatremia associated with these conditions,[60,61] hyponatremia occurs primarily because avid sodium and water reabsorption in the proximal tubule results in decreased delivery of filtrate to the diluting portion of the nephron and because slow flow through the collecting duct results in ADH-independent water reabsorption. The sodium avidity in the proximal tubule leads to a urine that is almost totally free of sodium. In SIADH, urine sodium is usually high since it reflects sodium intake. Urine sodium may be increased by diuretic use even in the face of volume contraction. Urine sodium in SIADH may be low if the patient is following a sodium-restricted diet or if nausea has limited oral intake. Measurement of T4, T3 resin uptake and thyroid-stimulating hormone will confirm the diagnosis of myxedema. Adrenal insufficiency should be suspected if hyponatremia is accompanied by hyperkalemia and an elevated BUN and creatinine. Often, however, the diagnosis of adrenal cortical or anterior pituitary insufficiency can be made only by measurement of basal and stimulated levels of adrenal and anterior pituitary hormones. A distinction between adrenal deficiency and other causes of SIADH can be made by the administration of physiologic doses of adrenal steroid hormones. Urinary diluting ability is somewhat improved in other forms of SIADH by the administration of mineralocorticoids, but only when very large doses are administered (20 mg of desoxycorticosterone acetate or 1 mg of aldosterone).[2]

A common misconception about SIADH is that urine osmolality must be greater than serum osmolality. When hypoosmolality is induced by excessive water intake in normal individuals, the urine is maximally dilute. If the urine osmolality is higher than maximally dilute, a water excreting defect is present even if urine osmolality does not exceed plasma osmolality. The inappropriately concentrated urine is characteristic of all hyponatremic states except psychogenic polydipsia and does not help in making the diagnosis of SIADH.

5. TREATMENT

5.1. Acute Treatment

The choice of treatment depends upon the severity of hyponatremia, the rapidity with which it developed, and the severity of clinical symptoms. Even if hyponatremia develops gradually, serum sodium levels below 110–115 mEq/liter are likely to cause severe and sometimes irreversible neurologic problems. Acute water intoxication is even less well tolerated. Arieff and

Guisado state that a drop in the serum sodium even to 125 mEq/liter or below within 24 hr is associated with frequent brain damage and a mortality rate of 50%.[3]

Rapid correction of hyponatremia with hypertonic saline is warranted whenever the serum sodium falls below 110 mEq/liter or when neurologic symptoms such as confusion, organic brain syndrome, or seizures are present at higher serum sodium. In these circumstances, restitution of blood osmolarity can be accomplished by giving furosemide, which results in production of urine that is approximately isotonic to plasma. The urine sodium should be measured hourly and the excreted sodium should be replaced milliequivalent for milliequivalent in the form of 3% saline (513 mEq/liter), as suggested by Hantman et al.[62] No free water should be given orally or intravenously until the serum sodium is above 115.

Treatment of SIADH in relatively asymptomatic patients, when the serum sodium is above 115 mEq/liter, can be accomplished by restricting water intake to 800 ml/day while continuing to provide dietary sodium to correct the sodium deficit that occurs during the development of hyponatremia before the patient reaches a steady state. Excess water is gradually decreased through insensible loss. The administration of normal saline will not correct the hyponatremia of SIADH because volume expansion decreases proximal sodium reabsorption, so that all the administered sodium is excreted.

Losses of water in excess of sodium losses can be induced with the use of an osmotic diuretic such as an infusion of urea.

5.2. Long-Term Treatment

The best long-term treatment of SIADH is to relieve the cause. Such treatment may be straightforward when it involves discontinuing a drug or replacing endocrine deficiency or treatment of the pulmonary infection. It is more difficult if SIADH is due to neurologic or neoplastic disease.

The definitive treatment of SIADH induced by tumor is to resect the tumor. Oat cell carcinoma of the lung is the most common tumor associated with SIADH. The tumor is not usually resectable, but reversal of SIADH by treatment of the tumor may occur if more effective chemotherapy for this tumor is developed. Tisher has reported a case of SIADH associated with adenocarcinoma of the lung that disappeared following resection of the tumor and reappeared prior to the development of clinically apparent metastases.[63]

When the primary disease cannot be treated, long-term treatment of SIADH with water restriction is possible if the patient adheres to it, but long-term water restriction usually proves impractical both because of habit and because thirst often accompanies SIADH.

Several drugs are available for the treatment of SIADH. The two most commonly used drugs are lithium and demeclocycline both of which affect the kidney's responsiveness to ADH.[64]

Although lithium does have a small effect on pituitary secretion of ADH in some people, in most, polyuria is a result of lithium-induced nephrogenic diabetes insipidus. Lithium acts in several ways, both ADH-dependent and -independent. When lithium is given to Brattleboro rats (ADH-deficient) their polyuria is increased. Lithium depresses sodium reabsorption in the proximal tubule while sodium chloride reabsorption in the ascending limb of the loop of the Henle is intact. The delivery of increased amounts of sodium chloride to the ascending limb results in increased reabsorption and increased generation of free water in the tubular fluid.[65]

Lithium is taken up by renal epithelial cells and uptake is stimulated by ADH. Lithium interferes with the water flow induced by exogenous ADH and to a lesser extent, the water flow induced by exogenous dibutyrl cAMP.[66] It appears to have an effect both proximal and distal to cAMP generation,[64] by noncompetitive inhibition of adenyl cyclase activity and impairment of the activity of a cAMP protein kinase.

Successful treatment of SIADH with 900 mg of lithium was reported in an adult whose fluid intake was 2 liters daily.[67] No change in urinary cAMP was noted during treatment. Baker et al. found serum levels of lithium of 0.3–0.6 mEq/liter to be effective in controlling SIADH in a child with a posterior fossa astrocytoma.[68] Such levels are below the therapeutic range for the treatment of manic depressive disease, in which levels of 0.6–1.5 mEq/liter are required. Known side effects of lithium include mild diarrhea and abdominal discomfort when the serum levels are 0.6–1.5 mEq/liter. When the serum lithium concentration is greater than 1.5 mEq/liter, severe neurologic problems, including drowsiness, coarse tremor, dysarthria, coma, and death, may occur. Lithium has also been noted to cause myocardial irritability.

Lithium has been replaced by demeclocycline, a tetracycline antibiotic, in the treatment of chronic SIADH. The abandonment of lithium in the treatment of SIADH followed a report by Forrest et al. in which two of three patients treated with lithium had neurologic side effects that required stopping the drug, even though lithium levels were between 0.4–1.2 mEq/liter.[69] None of the patients responded to lithium with a rise in serum sodium over a 3- to 5-day period. Baker et al.[68] had used lithium only after hyponatremia had been corrected with fluid restriction. In one case, a prompt water diuresis occurred after the administration of lithium while one patient was still hyponatremic.[67]

When demeclocycline was used for treatment of acne, it was noted that patients developed dose-related diabetes insipidus at 600 to 1200 mg/day. In the toad bladder, demeclocycline interferes with both ADH- and cAMP-induced water flow, suggesting that the site of action is at a point beyond cAMP generation. At very high doses, however, the inhibitory effect of demeclocycline on ADH-mediated water flow continues to increase. Since these higher doses do not increase the degree of inhibition of cAMP-mediated water flow, the drug must be acting in two separate sites. Demeclocycline binds to epithelial cell proteins, which are involved in mediating ADH- and cAMP-induced water flow.[64]

Most people with normal renal function who take demeclocycline develop dose-related nephrogenic diabetes insipidus, in contrast to only 12% of people taking lithium. Forrest et al. reported success in treating ten patients with severe SIADH (minimum urine osmolality 700–800 mOsm/kg) with demeclocycline, 600–1200 mg/day.[69] While these patients were being treated with demeclocycline urine osmolality fell to 275 mOsm/kg. Urinary sodium fell from 98 mEq/liter to 48 mEq/liter, body weight fell, and serum sodium rose from 122 mEq/liter to 139 mEq/liter. Demeclocycline begins to work within 5 days. Because it binds to blood proteins, demeclocycline can exert effects for as long as 10 days after it has been stopped. Other investigators have reported success with the use of this drug.[70–72] The most common side effects of demeclocycline are photosensitivity and superinfection related to its antibiotic properties. When used in patients with cirrhosis it can lead to reversible renal failure.[73,74] The drug should be used with caution in this group of patients.

Phenytoin and naloxone are drugs that decrease ADH secretion. Phenytoin suppresses ADH release from the pituitary gland, and it has been used for short-term treatment of patients with SIADH.[75] Fichman and Bethune noted improved handling of a water load in patients with SIADH pretreated with phenytoin.[76] They also noted that an improvement occurred in patients who had SIADH secondary to neurologic disease but not in patients with SIADH secondary to tumor, thereby possibly distinguishing ectopic ADH production from SIADH secondary to neurologic disease.[75] Tanay et al. report a patient with SIADH following basal skull fracture who developed intolerable side effects from demeclocycline and was then treated with phenytoin, which successfully controlled her SIADH for 8 months.[76]

Since the discovery of the β-endorphins and enkephalins, a role for these endogenous opioidlike peptides has been postulated. Miller noted that the administration of the narcotic antagonists oxilorphan and butorphanol leads to a decrease in maximum urinary concentration and a decrease in ADH response to hyperosmolality, but no change in renal response to exogenously administered ADH. These data suggest a direct effect on ADH release.[77] Miller and Moses have also reported success in treating patients with SIADH secondary to neurologic problems with narcotic antagonists.[78] As expected, treatment of SIADH secondary to bronchogenic carcinoma with narcotic antagonists was unsuccessful.

6. SUMMARY

SIADH is a syndrome in which a water excreting defect develops secondary to secretion of ADH inappropriately or in response to nonosmotic physiological stimuli. It occurs in the presence of tumors, in neurologic and pulmonary disease, in postoperative patients, and with the use of a wide array of drugs. The mainstay of treatment is water restriction. In emergency situations hypertonic saline may be necessary. Water restriction may be supplemented by the use of either drugs that cause nephrogenic diabetes insipidus or drugs that suppress ADH secretion.

ACKNOWLEDGMENT. I wish to thank Ms. Elaine Cuneo for excellent secretarial assistance in the preparation of the manuscript.

REFERENCES

1. Schwartz WB, Bennett W, Curelop S, et al: A syndrome of renal sodium loss and hyponatremia probably resulting from inappropriate secretion of antidiuretic hormone. *Am J Med* 23:529–542, 1957.
2. Bartter FC, Schwartz WB: The syndrome of inappropriate secretion of antidiuretic hormone. *Am J Med* 42:790–806, 1967.

3. Arieff AI, Guisado R: Effects on the central nervous system in hypernatremic and hyponatremic states. *Kidney Int* 10:104–116, 1976.

4. Beck LH: Hypouricemia in the syndrome of inappropriate secretion of antidiuretic hormone. *N Engl J Med* 301:528–530, 1979.

5. Biebisch G: Coupled ion and fluid transport in the kidney. *N Engl J Med* 287:913–919, 1972.

6. Cohen JJ, Hulter HN, Smithline N, et al: The critical role of the adrenal gland in the renal regulation of acid–base equilibrium during chronic hypotonic expansion. *J Clin Invest* 58:1201–1208, 1976.

7. Feig PH, McCurdy DK: The hypertonic state. *N Engl J Med* 297:1444–1454, 1977.

8. Robertson GL, Shelton RL, Athar S: The osmoregulation of vasopressin. *Kidney Int* 10:25–37, 1976.

9. DeFronzo RA, Goldberg M, Agus ZS: Normal diluting capacity in hyponatremic patients. *Ann Intern Med* 84:538–542, 1976.

10. Amatruda TT, Mulrow PJ, Gallagher JC, et al: Carcinoma of the lung with inappropriate antidiuresis. *N Engl J Med* 269:544–549, 1963.

11. Bower BF, Mason DM, Forsham PH, et al: Bronchogenic carcinoma with inappropriate antidiuretic activity in plasma and tumor. *N Engl J Med* 271:934–938, 1964.

12. Padfield PL, Morton JJ, Brown JJ, et al: Plasma arginine vasopressin in the syndrome of antidiuretic hormone excess associated with bronchogenic carcinoma. *Am J Med* 61:825–831, 1976.

13. Yamaji T, Ishibashi M, Katayama S: Nature of immunoreactive neurophysins in ectopic vasopressin-producing oat cell carcinoma of the lung. *J Clin Invest* 68:388–398, 1981.

14. Odell W, Wolfson A, Yoshimoto Y, et al: Ectopic peptide synthesis: A universal concommitant of neoplasia. *Trans Assoc Am Physicians* 90:204–227, 1977.

15. Fisher C, Ingram WR, Ranson SW: Diabetes insipidus and the neurohormonal control of water balance: A contribution to the structure and function of the hypothalamo-hypophysial system. Ann Arbor MI, Edwards Brothers, 1938.

16. Cobb WE: Endocrine management after pituitary surgery, in Post K, Jackson IMD, Reichlin S (eds): *The Pituitary Adenoma.* New York, Plenum Medical, 1980, pp 417–435.

17. Kaplan SL, Feigin RD: The syndrome of inappropriate secretion of antidiuretic hormone in children with bacterial meningitis. *J Pediatr* 92:758–761, 1978.

18. Moylan FMB, Herrin JT, Krishnamoorthy K, et al: Inappropriate antidiuretic hormone secretion in premature infants with cerebral injury. *Am J Dis Child* 132:399–402, 1978.

19. Goldberg M, Handler JS: Hyponatremia and renal wasting of sodium in patients with malfunction of the central nervous system. *N Engl J Med* 263:1037–1043, 1960.

20. Nelson PB, Sief SM, Maroon JC, et al: Hyponatremia in intracranial disease: Perhaps not the syndrome of inappropriate secretion of antidiuretic hormone. *Neurosurgery* 55:938–941, 1981.

21. Joynt RJ, Feibel JH, Sladek CM: Antidiuretic hormone levels in stroke patients. *Ann Neurosurg* 9:182–184, 1981.

22. Ludwig GD, Goldbert M: Hyponatremia in acute intermittent porphyria probably resulting from inappropriate secretion of antidiuretic hormone. *Ann NY Acad Sci* 104:710–734, 1963.

23. Hayes MA, Goldberg IS: Renal effects of anesthesia and operation mediated by endocrines. *Anesthesiology* 24:487–499, 1963.

24. Deutsch S, Goldberg M, Dripps RD: Postoperative hyponatremia with the inappropriate release of antidiuretic hormone. *Anesthesiology* 27:250–256, 1966.

25. Murdaugh HV, Sieker HO, Manfredi F: Effect of altered intrathoracic pressure on renal hemodynamics, electrolyte excretion and water clearance. *J Clin Invest* 238:834–842, 1959.

26. Kendler KS, Weitzman RE, Fisher DA: The effect of pain on plasma arginine vasopressin concentrations in man. *Clin Endocrinol* 8:89–94, 1978.

27. Philbin DM, Wilson NE, Sokoloski J, et al: Radioimmunoassay of antidiuretic hormone during morphine anaesthesia. *Can Anaesth Soc J* 23:290–295, 1976.

28. Weitzman RE, Fisher DA, Minick S, et al: β-Endorphin stimulates secretion of arginine vasopressin in vivo. *Endocrinology* 101:1643–1646, 1977.

29. Rosenow EC, Segar WE, Zehr JE: Inappropriate antidiuretic hormone secretion in pneumonia. *Mayo Clinic Proc* 47:169–174, 1972.

30. Rivers RPA, Forsling ML, Olver RP: Inappropriate secretion of antidiuretic hormone in infants with respiratory infections. *Arch Dis Child* 56:358–363, 1981.

31. Breuer R, Rubinow A: Inappropriate secretion of antidiuretic hormone and mycoplasma pneumonia infection. *Respiration* 42:217–219, 1981.

32. Vorherr H, Massry SG, Fallet R, et al: Antidiuretic principle in tuberculous lung tissue of a patient with pulmonary tuberculosis and hyponatremia. *Ann Intern Med* 72:383–387, 1970.

33. Derwerter FJ, Michelis M, Bloom ME, et al: Impaired water excretion of myxedema. *Am J Med* 51:41–53, 1971.

34. Skowsky WR, Kikuchi TA: The role of vasopressin in the impaired water excretion of myxedema. *Am J Med* 64:613–621, 1978.

35. Discala VA, Kinney MJ: Effects of myxedema on the renal diluting and concentrating mechanism. *Am J Med* 50:325–335, 1971.

36. Macaron C, Famuyiwa O: Hyponatremia of hypothyroidism. *Arch Intern Med* 138:820–822, 1978.

37. Agus ZS, Goldberg M: Role of antidiuretic hormone in the abnormal water diuresis of anterior hypopituitarism in man. *J Clin Invest* 50:1478–1489, 1971.

38. Ishikawa S, Schrier RW: Effect of arginine vasopressin antagonist on renal water excretion in glucocorticoid and mineralocorticoid deficient rats. *Kidney Int* 22:587–593, 1982.

39. Linshaw MA, Hipp T, Grusken A: Infantile psychogenic water drinking. *J Pediatr* 85:520–522, 1974.

40. Kohn B, Norman ME, Feldman H, et al: Hysterical polydipsia (compulsive water drinking) in children. *Am J Dis Child* 130:210–212, 1976.

41. Hariprasad MK, Eisinger RP, Nadler IM, et al: Hyponatremia in psychogenic polydipsia. *Arch Intern Med* 140:1639–1642, 1980.

42. Dubovsky SL, Grabon S, Berl T, et al: Syndrome of inappropriate secretion of antidiuretic hormone with exacerbated psychosis. *Ann Intern Med* 79:551–554, 1973.

43. Epstein FH, Levitin H, Glaser G, et al: Cerebral hyponatremia. *N Engl J Med* 265:513–518, 1961.

44. Whitaker MD, McArthur RG, Corenblum B, et al: Idiopathic sustained inappropriate secretion of ADH associated with hypertension and thirst. *Am J Med* 67:511–515, 1979.

45. Skowsky WR, Fisher DA: Intermittent idiopathic inappropriate vasopressin secretion in a child. *J Pediatr* 83:62–68, 1973.

46. Grumer HA, Derryberry W, Dubin A, et al: Idiopathic episodic, inappropriate secretion of antidiuretic hormone. *Am J Med* 32:954–963, 1962.

47. Waldvogel F, deSouza RC, Mach RS: Intoxication à l'eau due à une sécrétion inadéquate d'hormone antidiurétic (Syndrome de Schwartz–Bartter) d'origine idiopathique. *Schweiz Med Wochenschr* 97:929–932, 1967.

48. Weissman PN, Shenkman L, Gregerman RI: Chlorpropamide hyponatremia. *N Engl J Med* 284:65–71, 1971.

49. Fine D, Shedrovilzky H: Hyponatremia due to chlorpropamide. *Ann Intern Med* 72:83–87, 1970.

50. Zusman RM, Keiser HR, Handler JS: Inhibition of vasopressin stimulated prostaglandin E biosynthesis by chlorpropamide in the toad urinary bladder. *J Clin Invest* 60:1348–1353, 1977.
51. Davis FB, Davis PJ: Water metabolism in diabetes mellitus. *Am J Med* 70:210–214, 1981.
52. Moses AM, Miller M: Drug induced dilutional hyponatremia. *N Engl J Med* 291:1234–1239, 1974.
53. DeFronzo RA, Braine H, Colvin OM, et al: Water intoxication in man after cyclophosphamide therapy. Time course and relation to drug activation. *Ann Intern Med* 78:861–869, 1973.
54. Mir MA, Delamore IW: Hyponatraemia syndrome in acute myeloid leukemia. *Br Med J* 1:29–32, 1974.
55. Cutting HO: Inappropriate secretion of antidiuretic hormone secondary to vincristine therapy. *Am J Med* 51:269–271, 1971.
56. Peterson JC, Pollack RW, Mahoney JJ, et al: Inappropriate antidiuretic hormone secondary to a monoamine oxidase inhibitor. *J Am Med Assoc* 239:1422–1423, 1978.
57. Moses AM, Howenitz J, Van Germert M, et al: Clofibrate induced antidiuresis. *J Clin Invest* 51:535–542, 1973.
58. Fichman MP, Vorherr H, Kleeman CR, et al: Diuretic induced hyponatremia. *Ann Intern Med* 75:853–863, 1971.
59. Ashraf N, Lockaley R, Arieff AI: Thiazide induced hyponatremia with death or neurologic damage in outpatients. *Am J Med* 70:1163–1168, 1981.
60. Szatalowicz VL, Arnold PE, Chaimovitz C, et al: Radioimmunoassay of plasma arginine vasopressin in hyponatremic patients with congestive heart failure. *N Engl J Med* 305:263–266, 1981.
61. Bichet D, Szatalowicz VL, Chaimovitz C, et al: Role of vasopressin in abnormal water excretion in cirrhotic patients. *Ann Intern Med* 96:413–417, 1982.
62. Hantman D, Rossier B, Zohlman R, et al: Rapid correction of hyponatremia in the syndrome of inappropriate secretion of antidiuretic hormone. *Ann Intern Med* 78:870–875, 1973.
63. Tisher CC: Correction of an inappropriate ADH syndrome by tumor resection. *Arch Intern Med* 121:163–168, 1973.
64. Singer I, Forrest JN, Drug induced states of nephrogenic diabetes insipidus. *Kidney Int* 10:82–95, 1976.
65. Decaux G, Unger J, Brimioulle S, et al: Hyponatremia in the syndrome of inappropriate secretion of antidiuretic hormone. *J Am Med Assoc* 247:471–474, 1982.
66. Forrest JN, Cohen AD, Torretti J, et al: On the mechanism of lithium induced diabetes insipidus in man and the rat. *J Clin Invest* 53:1115–1123, 1974.
67. White MG, Fetner CD: Treatment of the syndrome of inappropriate secretion of antidiuretic hormone with lithium carbonate. *N Engl J Med* 292:390–392, 1975.
68. Baker RS, Hurley RM, Feldman W: Treatment of recurrent syndrome of inappropriate secretion of antidiuretic hormone with lithium. *J Pediatr* 90:480–481, 1977.
69. Forrest JN, Cox M, Hong C, et al: Superiority of demeclocycline over lithium in the treatment of chronic syndrome of inappropriate secretion of antidiuretic hormone. *N Engl J Med* 298:173–177, 1978.
70. Graze K, Molitch ME, Post K: Chronic demeclocycline therapy in the syndrome of inappropriate ADH secretion due to brain tumor. *J Neurosurg* 47:933–936, 1977.
71. Cherill DA, Stote RM, Birge JR, et al: Demeclocycline treatment in the syndrome of inappropriate antidiuretic hormone secretion. *Ann Intern Med* 83:654–656, 1975.
72. DeTroyer A, Demanet JC: Correction of antidiuresis by demeclocycline. *N Eng J Med* 293:915–918, 1975.

73. DeTroyer A, Pilloy W, Broeckaert I, et al: Demeclocycline treatment of water retention in cirrhosis. *Ann Intern Med* 85:336–337, 1976.
74. Oster JR, Epstein M, Ulano HB: Deterioration of renal function with demeclocycline administration. *Curr Ther Rep* 20:794–801, 1976.
75. Fichman MP, Bethune JE: The role of adrenocorticoids in the inappropriate antidiuretic hormone syndrome. *Ann Intern Med* 68:806–820, 1968.
76. Tanay A, Yust I, Peresecenschi G, et al: Long-term treatment of the syndrome of inappropriate antidiuretic hormone secretion with phenytoin. *Ann Intern Med* 90:50–52, 1979.
77. Miller M: Role of endogenous opioids in neurohypophysial function of man. *J Clin Endocrinol Metab* 50:1016–1020, 1980.
78. Miller M, Moses AM: Clinical states due to alteration of ADH release and action, in: *Neurohypophysis: International Conference,* Key Biscayne, Florida. Basel, S. Karger, 1977, pp 153–166.

10

TREATMENT OF SICKLE CELL ANEMIA WITH dDAVP

Franklin H. Epstein, Robert M. Rosa, and H. Franklin Bunn

1. INTRODUCTION

The recurrent painful crises of sickle cell anemia, a major cause of morbidity and disability in this disease, result from what has been termed "a vicious cycle of erythrostasis."[1] In the hypoxic environment of the capillary bed, hemoglobin S is deoxygenated and red cells sickle owing to the formation of tactoids, or crystallike fibers, from the polymerization of deoxyhemoglobin S molecules. Resistance to blood flow is thereby increased, passage of red cells through capillaries is further delayed, and more deoxygenation and sickling ensue.

The tendency of cells containing sickle hemoglobin to assume the sickle shape depends primarily on the concentration of intracellular deoxyhemoglobin S. Since human red cells behave as osmometers, it follows that sickling may be enhanced by an increase in the concentration of sodium in plasma, and decreased in a hypotonic medium. The increased sickling of erythrocytes observed in a hypertonic solution resembling that of the renal medulla has been invoked as a possible explanation for the reduction of blood flow to the renal medulla in patients with sickle cell anemia, with consequent diminution in renal concentrating ability and predisposition to papillary necrosis. Con-

Franklin H. Epstein and Robert M. Rosa • Charles A. Dana Research Institute, Harvard–Thorndike Laboratory, and Department of Medicine, Beth Israel Hospital, Harvard Medical School, Boston, Massachusetts 02115. H. Franklin Bunn • Hematology Division, Department of Medicine, Brigham and Women's Hospital, Harvard Medical School, Boston, Massachusetts 02115.

versely, a reduction in plasma sodium might be expected to produce swelling of red cells, to reduce the intracellular concentration of deoxyhemoglobin S, and therefore to reduce the tendency to sickle.

The influence of cell swelling on the tendency of red blood cells to sickle should be amplified considerably by two interesting properties of sickle hemoglobin. The first is that the oxygen affinity of hemoglobin S is inversely proportional to its concentration. Dilution of the red cell contents therefore not only should reduce the concentration of hemoglobin but will further increase the oxygen affinity of hemoglobin S, thus decreasing the percentage of hemoglobin in the deoxy form.[2] A second interesting feature has to do with the small, finite time required for molecules of deoxyhemoglobin S to polymerize into fibers and for these fibers to align to form a crystalline phase. This is called the delay time of gelation. The delay time of gelation of deoxyhemoglobin S is said to be inversely proportional to the 30th power of the concentration of deoxyhemoglobin S. This exponential relationship provides enormous leverage. As pointed out by Eaton, Hofrichter, and Ross,[3,4] sickling will produce tissue ischemia only if the delay time of gelation is shorter than the capillary transit time. If the time taken for red cells to assume the sickle shape is prolonged until the cells emerge from the venous end of the capillary, the vicious circle of erythrostasis that is the basis of sickle cell crisis might be avoided.

Although oral and intravenous hydration has long been a standby in the treatment of sickle cell crisis, even rapid intravenous hydration with fluids low in sodium is generally ineffective in reducing serum sodium very much below normal, because of the considerable ability of normal kidneys to excrete a water load. Though patients with sickle cell anemia are notoriously unable to concentrate the urine, their diluting ability is usually unimpaired. Intravenous or oral water loads are therefore excreted rapidly without appreciable dilution of the serum sodium. The development of a long-acting derivative of arginine vasopressin with potent antidiuretic properties, 1-desamino-8-D-arginine vasopressin (dDAVP), has made it possible for the first time to produce at will a controlled state of hyponatremia. This is accomplished by asking patients to drink from 3500 to 4000 ml of water daily and insuring that their kidneys are constantly under the influence of antidiuretic hormone (ADH) by administering 0.4 ml of dDAVP intranasally four times a day.[5]

We have examined the effects of this regimen in four patients with recurrent disabling sickle cell crises. The patients were selected because during the six months to one year preceding the trial they had been incapacitated by recurrent painful crises. They usually required hospital admission approximately monthly for painful episodes requiring intravenous fluids and narcotics for relief. It should be appreciated that these individuals represent only a small subset of the general population of homozygous sickle cell anemia patients, since in most patients sickle cell crisis occurs less frequently. The objective was to decrease serum sodium at the rate of 5–8 mEq/liter per day to a level of approximately 125 mEq/liter. In most patients the regimen of fluids and dDAVP had to be supplemented with diuretics (100 mg of chlorothiazide or 40 mg of furosemide daily) when they left the hospital, in order to compensate for increased salt taken in the diet at home. Transient muscle cramps were experienced by two patients, but there were no central nervous system symptoms and no disturbances in neurological or cognitive function. The electroencephalogram remained normal in all patients.

2. RESULTS

2.1. Effect of Chronic Hyponatremia on Mean Corpuscular Hemoglobin Concentration

Figure 1 illustrates that chronic hyponatremia was in fact effective in decreasing mean corpuscular hemoglobin concentration. The fall in intracellular hemoglobin concentration was not significantly different from that

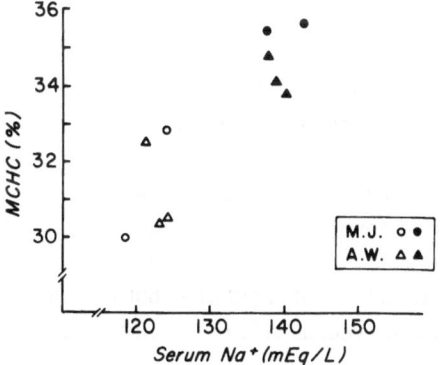

FIGURE 1. Effect of serum sodium on mean corpuscular hemoglobin concentration (MCHC) in two patients with sickle cell anemia. Solid symbols represent MCHC when the patients were normonatremic; open symbols represent MCHC when they were hyponatremic.

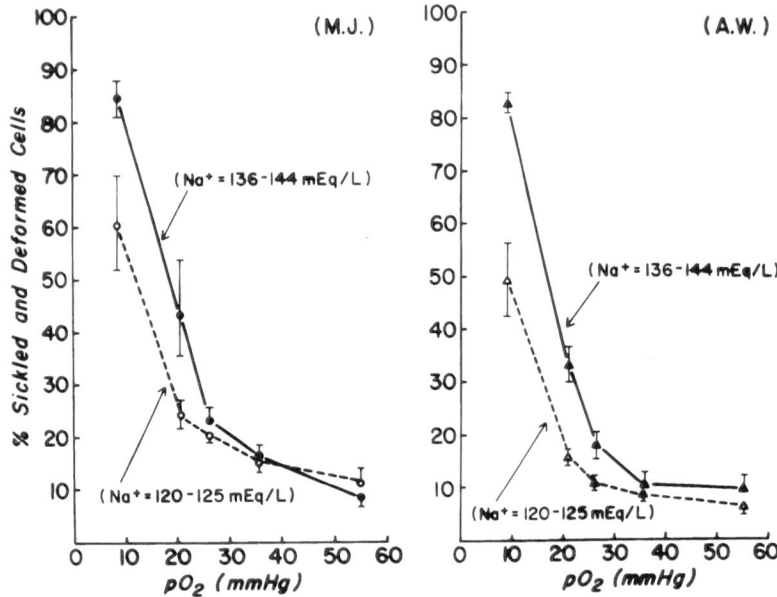

FIGURE 2. Effect of serum sodium on formation of sickled and deformed cells at varying oxygen tensions (Po₂) in two patients with sickle cell anemia.

predicted on the assumption that the red cells acted as perfect osmometers. Thus, at least in these patients, there appears to be little or no tendency of human red blood cells to counter-regulate their size in response to hypoosmotic swelling, as is the case in nucleated red blood cells of birds or fish.

2.2. Effect of Hyponatremia on Percentage of Sickle Cells at Varying Oxygen Tensions of Blood

Chronic hyponatremia was effective in reducing the percentage of sickled or deformed cells in the blood (Figure 2). In the two patients illustrated, the effect, as expected, was minimal at oxygen tensions close to those at the arterial end of capillaries, but was clearly apparent at the low Po_2 anticipated on the venous side of capillaries in organs with low blood flow.

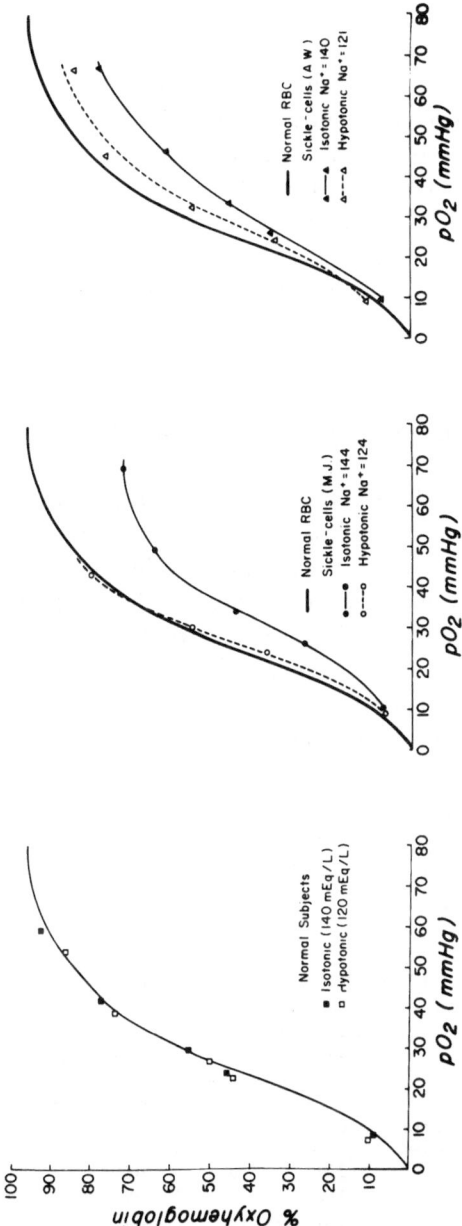

FIGURE 3. Effect of serum sodium on oxyhemoglobin dissociation curve in a volunteer with normal hemoglobin and in two patients with sickle cell anemia.

2.3. Effect on Oxygen Affinity of Hemoglobin S

The effect of hyponatremia on the oxygen affinity of the blood of two patients is illustrated in Figure 3. As shown previously by others, the oxygen dissociation curve of patients with sickle cell anemia is shifted to the right, i.e., at any given P_{O_2}, more hemoglobin is in the deoxy form than is true of normal blood.[2] When these patients were rendered hyponatremic, the oxygen dissociation curve shifted to the left, to or toward the normal curve. Changes in serum sodium do not alter the oxygen dissociation curve of normal red cells.[2,5]

2.4. Effect of Hyponatremia on Prevention of Sickle Cell Crises

The clinical effects of chronic sustained hyponatremia are seen in Table I. In all patients the occurrence of painful sickle cell crises was greatly reduced or completely eliminated when they were hyponatremic. In addition, the patients reported that generalized aching in the muscle joints and abdomen was less pronounced after hyponatremia was induced than it had been before therapy was initiated. When serum sodium fell below 120 mmoles/liter, however, anorexia and fatigue developed in all patients. Because prolonged treatment with dDAVP has been reported to stimulate the production of Factor VIII in some patients with hemophilia, we measured plasma levels of Factor VIII antigen, and found them to be twice the normal value. No episodes of spontaneous thrombosis or phlebitis occurred.

A practical difficulty encountered in long-term outpatient treatment, however, was the tendency of serum sodium to rise despite continued use of

TABLE I. Effect of Hyponatremia on the
Incidence of Sickle Cell Crisis

Case	Normal sodium		Hyponatremia	
	No. of days	No. of crises	No. of days	No. of crises
1	270	6	100	1
2	214	7	190	0
3	416	14	569	3
4	120	5	130	0

TABLE II. Effect of Acute Induction of Hyponatremia on the Duration of Sickle Cell Crises

	Conventional treatment			Induction of hyponatremia		
Case	No. of crises	Duration[a] (days)	Sodium[a] (mmoles/liter)	No. of crises	Duration[a] (days)	Sodium[b] (mmoles/liter)
1	6	18 ± 6	140 ± 1	2	9 ± 4	136 → 120
2	7	16 ± 3	143 ± 1	3	4 ± 3	139 → 125
3	14	7 ± 1	140 ± 2	2	4 ± 0	140 → 122
TOTAL	27	11.8 ± 2.3		7	5.4 ± 4[c]	

[a] Values are reported as the mean ± SE.
[b] Figures before and after the arrow denote sodium concentrations before and after hyponatremia was induced.
[c] $p < 0.01$ by Student's t-test for group mean.

dDAVP. This may have been due to the increased intake of solute, including both salt and protein, when patients left the hospital. Adults with sickle-cell anemia have permanent impairment of renal concentrating ability, with a maximum urinary solute concentration in the neighborhood of 350–400 mOsm/kg water, about one-third the normal value. Obligatory urinary losses of water, even under the influence of maximal amounts of ADH, are therefore about three times normal, and the effect of an increase in solute intake in exacerbating urinary volume is proportionally increased. Continuous self-discipline is necessary to maintain a high fluid intake. An additional factor, the possible role of increased renal prostaglandin production in counteracting the antidiuretic effect of dDAVP, remains to be investigated.

2.5. Dilutional Hyponatremia in the Treatment of Acute Sickle Cell Crisis

Throughout the study there were nine episodes of sickle cell crisis in the four patients, but only two of these crises occurred when the patients were hyponatremic. The other seven occurred when the patients' serum sodium became normal at home. When crises occurred while the patients were normonatremic, hyponatremia was induced by intravenous administration of 5% dextrose and water and intranasal administration of dDAVP. The duration of the sickle cell crisis was significantly shortened (Table II). Lowering serum sodium by 7–8 mEq/liter per day until it reached a level of 120–125 mEq/liter approximately halved the duration of crises in comparison with crises treated by conventional means before admission to the study. No untoward symptoms were observed when serum sodium was lowered in this manner.

2.6. Effect of Hyponatremia on Red Blood Cell Survival

In one patient, the red cell survival time was studied by chromium labeling when the serum sodium was normal and after hyponatremia had been induced for 3 months. The half-time of survival was significantly prolonged in the hyponatremic state, suggesting that hemolysis owing to intravascular sickling had been substantially diminished.

3. DISCUSSION

Sickling of erythrocytes depends on the polymerization of deoxyhemoglobin S within the cell. The time required for this event to occur varies widely with the experimental conditions. According to Hofrichter et al., the delay time of gelation of purified deoxyhemoglobin S is inversely proportional to the 30th power of the deoxyhemoglobin S concentration.[3] Therefore, relatively small decreases in mean corpuscular hemoglobin concentration, produced by a decline in serum sodium like those observed in our patients, should cause substantial delays in the rate of sickle cell formation.[4] A decrease in serum sodium to the range of 120–125 mmoles/liter would be associated with a 30- to 100-fold increase in the time required for gelation. This delay may well be long enough to allow red cells containing sickle hemoglobin to pass through capillary beds before sickling occurs, thereby reducing erythrostasis in small blood vessels and decreasing the frequency and duration of painful crises.

There are other reasons why a long-term decrease in serum sodium should reduce sickling of erythrocytes in vivo. During hyponatremia, the affinity of sickle hemoglobin for oxygen is increased, so that at any given partial oxygen pressure less of the hemoglobin is in the deoxy form, which is required for polymerization.[2] In addition, hydration of sickle cells appears to reduce the rigidity of irreversibly sickled forms.[6]

Although severe hyponatremia may be associated with a variety of distrubances in function of the central nervous system, including hyporeflexia, impaired mentation, and convulsions, no untoward effects were seen in the three patients studied, except that mild muscle cramps occurred when the serum sodium was reduced rapidly below 120 mmoles/liter. We would be reluctant to recommend prolonged reduction in serum sodium below 120 mmoles/liter, since the effects of this degree of severe and prolonged hyponatremia on brain function are not known. Special precautions will be necessary in the application of this therapy to the prevention of sickle cell crisis in children, since hyponatremia may be more likely to predispose them to convulsions. The practical difficulties in adjusting serum sodium during long-term treatment and the potential hazards of water intoxication emphasize that dilution hyponatremia should not be applied indiscriminately, but should be reserved at present for severely afflicted patients who can be studied in a properly controlled and carefully scrutinized setting.

4. SUMMARY

Chronic hyponatremia has been induced in four patients with severe sickle cell anemia. Therapy has resulted in a corresponding reduction in mean corpuscular hemoglobin concentration and a decreased degree of sickling, as determined by morphological criteria and by an increase in oxygen affinity. Sustained treatment appears to reduce the frequency of crises, and acute induction of hyponatremia appears to shorten their duration.

It must be strongly emphasized that these studies are preliminary and involved patients who served as their own historical controls. Furthermore, sickle cell anemia is a relatively common disease that has a long and often variable course. Nonetheless, the consistency of the clinical observations and hematological measurements is encouraging. They warrant, we believe, a larger and carefully controlled study to determine the efficacy and safety of induced hyponatremia in the prevention and treatment of sickle cell crisis. In addition, the efficacy of other measures designed to reduce either the concentration of deoxyhemoglobin S in red cells or its rate of molecular aggregation may be inhanced by even mild hyponatremia. Poised at the edge of painful crisis, these patients may derive crucial benefit from a modest and easily produced long-term increase in the volume of their red cells.

ACKNOWLEDGMENTS. The research on which this chapter is based was supported in part by grants (AM-17199, AM-27155, AM-07026, AM-17148, and HL-16927) from the United States Public Health Service; by a grant (RR-01032) from the General Clinical Research Center Branch, Division of Research Resources; by the Howard Hughes Medical Institute; by the William F. Milton Fund, Harvard Medical School; and by Ferring Pharmaceuticals.

REFERENCES

1. Ham TH, Castle WB: Relation of increased hypotonic fragility and of erythrostasis to the mechanism of hemolysis in certain anemias. *Trans Assoc Am Physicians* 55:127–132, 1940.
2. May A, Huehns ER: The concentration dependence of the oxygen affinity of haemoglobin S. *Br J Haematol* 30:317–335, 1975.
3. Hofrichter J, Ross PD, Eaton WA: Kinetics and mechanism of deoxyhemoglobin S gelation: A new approach to understanding sickle cell disease. *Proc Natl Acad Sci USA* 71:4864–4868, 1974.
4. Eaton WA, Hofrichter J, Ross PD: Delay time of gelation: A possible determinant of clinical severity in sickle cell disease. *Blood* 47:621–627, 1976.
5. Rosa RM, Bierer BE, Thomas R, et al: A study of induced hyponatremia in the prevention and treatment of sickle-cell crisis. *N Engl J Med* 303:1138–1143, 1980.
6. Clark MR, Mohandas N, Shohet SB: Deformability of oxygented irreversibly sickled cells. *J Clin Invest* 65:189–196, 1980.

11

dDAVP IN VON WILLEBRAND'S DISEASE AND IN MODERATELY SEVERE HEMOPHILIA A

Jeanne M. Lusher and A. Indira Warrier

1. INTRODUCTION

This chapter concerns the use of the vasopressin analogue 1-desamino-8-D-arginine vasopressin (dDAVP) in the treatment of von Willebrand's disease and mild or moderate hemophilia A. Both of these hereditary bleeding disorders are characterized by a subnormal amount of Factor VIII (F VIII) activity. Hemophilia A, which is inherited as a sex-linked recessive trait, and thus affects males almost exclusively, is characterized by bleeding into joints and muscles. Affected individuals have low levels of F VIII procoagulant activity (F VIII:C), but normal or increased amounts of the other two components of the F VIII system, F VIII related antigen (F VIII:RAg) and von Willebrand factor (vWF).[1] While most individuals with hemophilia A have the severe form of the disease, with no detectable F VIII:C on assay, in some families affected males have a mild or moderate deficiency of F VIII:C, with values being approximately 2–15% of normal.

Jeanne M. Lusher and A. Indira Warrier • Children's Hospital of Michigan, Detroit, Michigan 48201.

While severity varies considerably, affected individuals characteristically have prolonged bleeding times, mucous membrane bleeding, and excessive bleeding following dental extractions or other surgical procedures.[1,2] The situation in vWD is somewhat more complicated than that in hemophilia, in that a large number of vWD variants have now been recognized. In addition to quantitative variants, qualitative variants occur in which an abnormal (and often nonfunctional) molecular form of F VIII is produced.[2-12]

How are these two disorders treated, and where does dDAVP come in to the treatment schema? Until 1967, bleeding episodes in individuals with hemophilia or vWD were treated with whole plasma, as no one had developed an effective way of separating F VIII from plasma. Dr. Judith Pool's discovery in that year of a simple method for preparing cryoprecipitates from single units of plasma was a tremendous advance. Shortly thereafter, effective methods for preparing lyophilized F VIII concentrates from large pools of plasma were developed. The availability of these concentrated F VIII preparations greatly improved the lives of individuals with hemophilia and vWD. For the first time, beginning in late 1967, outpatient treatment for acute bleeding episodes could be carried out, using cryoprecipitates. If a young man with hemophilia began bleeding into a joint, it no longer meant several days of hospitalization; rather, he could get an infusion of concentrated F VIII and go home. The availability of F VIII concentrates also made elective surgical procedures possible. In addition, home treatment programs became a reality in the 1970s. These self-infusion programs proved to have many benefits, not only medical, but socioeconomic and psychological as well. From a strictly medical standpoint, prompt treatment of early joint bleeding at home should greatly lessen the incidence of disabling chronic joint disease.

While the availability of F VIII concentrates has greatly improved the lives of individuals with hemophilia and vWD, and has no doubt lessened the incidence of chronic hemophiliac arthropathy and crippling deformities, these concentrates are not without risk. In the individual who receives blood products, especially those components prepared from large numbers of plasma donors, the hepatitis risk (particularly for non-A, non-B hepatitis) is still quite high.[13-27] In those who develop hepatitis, long-term sequelae may include chronic active hepatitis or chronic hepatitis.[26,27]

For at least some of these individuals—those with mild or moderate hemophilia A and those with classical vWD or quantitative vWD variants—

there now appears to be an alternative to treatment with blood products, namely, dDAVP.

2. HISTORICAL ASPECTS

In 1903 Vosburgh and Richards noted an acceleration of the whole blood clotting time in dogs after giving adrenalin.[28] Despite a number of studies, the reasons for this remained obscure for over 50 years. The first clue to the underlying mechanism was the discovery by Marciniakøwna in 1957 that injection of adrenalin into rabbits was followed by a rise in F VIII activity.[29] This observation was later confirmed in man,[30] and it was shown that the rise in F VIII also occurred in individuals with mild hemophilia and in those with vWD. Brisk exercise produced a similar rise in F VIII activity, both in normals and in mild hemophiliacs, and this also seemed to be mediated by adrenalin release.[31] The effect of a single stimulus lasted only a few hours, but repeated responses could be obtained,[32] and it seemed that some clinical use could be made of this finding. However, the side effects of adrenalin were unpleasant, and vigorous exercise was not always appropriate in a bleeding patient, so little progress was made beyond occasional attempts to improve the yield of F VIII by treating or exercising blood donors.

Meanwhile, in Europe other stimuli were investigated. Mannucci et al.[33] and Cash et al.[34] tested other vasoactive drugs and found that vasopressin also raised F VIII activity. Again, unfortunately, the side effects were unpleasant, but then it was found that the symptomless analogue, dDAVP, worked as well.[35] Like all the other stimuli tested, dDAVP also briefly enhanced fibrinolytic activity. In 1977, Mannucci and colleagues reported the first clinical trials with dDAVP in the management of posttraumatic bleeding in mild hemophilia and vWD, and it appeared that the drug was useful in management.[35]

3. dDAVP: MECHANISM OF ACTION

What do we know about this drug and its mechanism of action on the clotting system? When given either intranasally or intravenously, dDAVP results in a short-term increase in plasminogen activator, and in all components of the F VIII system. Its mechanism of action is not known with certainty, but it has been postulated that dDAVP acts through release of a second messenger, probably from the central nervous system, which results in release of F VIII from its vessel wall endothelial cell storage sites. The rise in all components of the F VIII system produced by dDAVP appears so rapidly that increased synthesis is unlikely to account for it, and the endogenous release of autologous F VIII appears more likely.[11,35,36]

4. CLINICAL TRIALS AND OBSERVATIONS WITH dDAVP IN EUROPE

In the first reported clinical trials, Mannucci and colleagues used dDAVP intravenously, infusing the drug over a 5-min period. In these patients, who were undergoing surgery, the fibrinolytic inhibitor tranexamic acid was also used. Surgical procedures done with dDAVP coverage included extraction of permanent teeth, lymph node biopsy, tonsillectomy, cholecystectomy, and thoracotomy with lung biopsy. Dosage of dDAVP was 0.4–0.5 mg/kg per dose, and doses were repeated every 12 hr. Often the response diminished somewhat with repeated doses, suggesting that stores were being depleted. These workers also reported that dDAVP was also completely devoid of the unpleasant vasoactive and gastrointestinal side effects of the other vasopressin derivatives. Furthermore, they noted that while dDAVP has a powerful antidiuretic effect in patients with diabetes insipidus, no water overload occurred in individuals who did not have diabetes insipidus. In Mannucci's vWD and hemophilia subjects undergoing surgery, there was no restriction of water intake, and intravenous fluids were given as usual during anesthesia and postoperatively.[35]

4.1. Effect of dDAVP on Bleeding Time

In Mannucci's early studies, he noted that the bleeding time was not corrected in vWD subjects by dDAVP, and in fact that the bleeding time was not corrected in these subjects even after infusion of cryoprecipitates.[36] It is noteworthy, however, that most other groups have reported normalization or near-normalization of the bleeding time in vWD with either cryoprecipitate or dDAVP,[11,37-40] and it now appears that the bleeding time will return to normal in some types of vWD (classical vWD and quantitative variants), but not in others (qualitative variants in which an abnormal, nonfunctional form of F VIII is produced).

4.2. Clinicopharmacologic Studies

Some of the more recent studies of Mannucci and colleagues have been directed at providing clinicopharmacologic information relevant to the use of dDAVP in persons with vWD and mild hemophilia. In normal subjects a variety of doses were tried, and intravenous dDAVP was found to produce its maximal response in a dosage of 0.3 μg/kg body weight. When it was administered intranasally, a larger dose had to be given, and the increase in F VIII was less (approximately twofold, versus threefold with intravenous administration). Mannucci et al. also studied individuals with mild hemophilia A and with mild and moderate vWD, and they found similar percentage increases in both F VIII:C and F VIII:RAg, although the percent increase in F VIII:RAg was not as great as that in F VIII:C in any of the groups.[41]

After a single intravenous dose of dDAVP, serial assays were performed and the half-disappearance time was calculated. In healthy subjects the maximum rise was at 90 min and the half-disappearance time of F VIII:C was 4.5–5 hr. While similar findings were noted in vWD subjects, for some unknown reason the half-disappearance time was even longer in subjects with mild hemophilia A. The half-disappearance time of F VIII:RAg was 8–10 hr in all three groups.[41]

Mannucci also studied the response of normal subjects to five daily infusions of dDAVP. Following the second and third doses, the response of both F VIII:C and F VIII:RAg was significantly reduced compared with the first response, suggesting that stores were being depleted. There was a tendency to recover the initial response by the fourth day.[41]

5. UNITED STATES EXPERIENCE WITH dDAVP

In addition to the European experience, dDAVP has been used successfully in Japan,[6] in Australia,[38] and in the United States. dDAVP for this purpose is still considered investigational in the United States. Thus, we had to obtain an investigational new drug number from the Food and Drug Administration in order to use the drug.

5.1. Materials and Methods

5.1.1. Intranasal dDAVP

dDAVP for intranasal use was that commercially available from Ferring Pharmaceuticals and marketed for use as an antidiuretic hormone for individuals with diabetes insipidus. This material contains 0.1 mg dDAVP per ml, and it was slowly administered as an intranasal drip. The dosage of dDAVP used was 2–4 µg/kg body weight.

5.1.2. Intravenous dDAVP

dDAVP for intravenous use was obtained from Ferring Pharmaceuticals, and later from Revlon-Armour, when that company obtained the U.S. rights to the drug. The parenteral form contains 4 µg/ml, and it was given in a dosage of 0.2 or 0.3 µg/kg body weight. As recommended by Mannucci et al.,[41] the drug was mixed with 50 ml of normal saline solution immediately prior to use, and was injected slowly over a period of 15 min.

5.1.3. Subjects Studied in Michigan

Subjects consisted of 24 individuals with vWD, seven with mild to moderate hemophilia A, and three normal controls. Informed consent was obtained from all study subjects, and the study protocol was approved by the hospital's research and investigations committee. Of the 24 vWD subjects, two (ages 5 and 15 years) had severe vWD, while 22 had mild or moderate vWD. None of the latter group had an abnormal form of F VIII:RAg as demonstrated by crossed immunoelectrophoresis. All but two of the vWD subjects were not bleeding when given dDAVP for the first time. Six of the mild to moderate vWD subjects received dDAVP again immediately prior to tonsillectomy, nasal polypectomy, dental extractions, or other oral surgical procedures. Two other subjects were given dDAVP at the time of excessive menstrual bleeding.

The seven subjects with mild to moderate hemophilia A had baseline F VIII:C values of 0.02–0.12 U/ml (2–12%). Four of these individuals were not bleeding when first studied, while three were given dDAVP for treatment of acute hemarthroses or muscle hemorrhage on one or more occasions. One boy received dDAVP just prior to an oral surgical procedure.

5.1.4. Methods and Tests Performed

Pulse rate and blood pressure determinations were recorded on all subjects immediately before dDAVP administration, and at 15, 30, and 60 min post-dDAVP. All subjects had normal baseline values for pulse rate and blood pressure. No attempt was made to restrict fluid intake.

F VIII:C was assayed by the one-stage method.[42] F VIII:RAg was measured by a modification of the Laurell technique (method of Zimmerman et al.[43]), and ristocetin cofactor activity (F VIII:RCof or vWF) was measured by the macroscopic agglutination method using formalin-fixed, washed platelets.[44] Fibrinolytic activity (plasminogen activator) was measured by the euglobulin lysis time.[45] Bleeding times, done on vWD subjects, were performed by the modified Ivy technique, using a template.[46,47]

5.2. Observations and Results

5.2.1. Intranasal dDAVP

The commercially available intranasal preparation of dDAVP is quite dilute, necessitating that a volume of 2 ml be given. Some of this large volume of material was lost by swallowing in several subjects. Nevertheless, the majority had a marked increase in F VIII activity following dDAVP. Thirteen vWD subjects were given dDAVP intranasally. One, a 15-year-old girl with severe vWD, had no rise in F VIII. The other 12, who had mild or moderate vWD, all exhibited an increase in F VIII:C (average increase 200% over baseline values). Ten of 12 had an increase in F VIII:RAg (average increase

40% over baseline values), while 9 of 12 had an increase in F VIII:RCof (average 50% over baseline values). The pre- and post-dDAVP bleeding times of four vWD subjects were measured. The only subject who had a prolonged baseline bleeding time showed a normal bleeding time 90 min post-dDAVP, but by 3 hr post-dDAVP it was again prolonged.

Two vWD subjects who had shown a good response to dDAVP when not bleeding later underwent extractions of permanent teeth immediately following intranasal dDAVP. Neither had any unusual bleeding. Both subjects were given the antifibrinolytic agent epsilon amino caproic acid (EACA) for several days postextraction, as is our usual practice for persons with hemophilia or vWD. A third vWD subject who had mucous membrane bleeding at the time of intranasal dDAVP administration ceased bleeding within 20 min following dDAVP.

Three individuals with moderate hemophilia A (baseline VIII:C values of 0.02, 0.07, and 0.07 U/ml) were given dDAVP intranasally. Two had increases in all components of the F VIII system post-dDAVP, while the third (who reported swallowing much of the dose) did not. One of the boys, who had previously exhibited a good response, later underwent an oral surgical procedure, intranasal dDAVP being given 15 min preoperatively and EACA postoperatively. No unusual bleeding occurred during or after the procedure.

5.2.2. Intravenous dDAVP

When intravenous dDAVP (0.2–0.3 μg/kg) was given to three normal subjects, a rapid rise in all F VIII activities was noted. Maximum VIII:C (320% over baseline) and VIII:RAg (217% over baseline) levels were observed at 3 hrs and all three subjects had persistently elevated levels at 6 hr post-dDAVP. All eleven individuals with mild or moderate vWD who were given a single intravenous dose of 0.2 μg/kg also exhibited a marked sustained rise in all components of the F VIII system, with peak VIII:C values averaging 202% over baseline, peak VIII:RAg values averaging 152% over baseline, and VIII:RCof averaging 121% over baseline.

One child with vWD underwent tonsillectomy, one underwent nasal polypectomy, and a third underwent dental extractions 30 min after intravenous administration of dDAVP. Excessive bleeding did not occur in any of them. Each of two vWD subjects who had severe menorrhagia at the time of intravenous dDAVP administration exhibited shortening of the bleeding time to normal (within 15 min) and marked lessening of menstrual bleeding within a few hours.

Three individuals with moderate hemophilia A (baseline values 0.03–0.12 U/ml) were given intravenous dDAVP. Each exhibited a rise in all F VIII components, with VIII:C values increasing an average of 300%. One boy received intravenous dDAVP for treatment of acute hemarthroses on three separate occasions, while another subject received dDAVP for acute hemarthrosis on one occasion and for two episodes of soft tissue hemorrhage. Both subjective and objective improvement were noted in all six bleeding episodes.

5.2.3. Untoward Side Effects

No deleterious side effects were noted in any of the 34 subjects who received dDAVP in either form (intranasally or intravenously). None had an elevation in pulse rate or blood pressure over their normal baseline values. None developed headache or other complaints.

None of the subjects had a shortening of euglobulin lysis time to less than 60 min in blood samples obtained 30 and 90 min post-dDAVP.

6. DISCUSSION

Despite regulations that all blood products be tested for hepatitis B surface antigen, the use of cryoprecipitates and lyophilized F VIII concentrates is still associated with a definite risk of transmission of hepatitis virus.[13–27] Thus, an alternative to the use of blood products for treatment of hemophilia and vWD would have distinct merit. For at least some individuals with hemophilia A and vWD, the vasopressin analogue dDAVP appears to be a safe and reasonably effective alternative to treatment with blood products.

6.1. Intranasal versus Intravenous Administration

In our own studies, as well as those of Mannucci et al.,[41] a larger and more consistent rise in F VIII was observed when dDAVP was given intravenously. Thus, for a more predictable and maximal rise in F VIII activities, the intravenous route would seem preferable to the intranasal route. However, the intranasal route may prove sufficient for minor bleeding episodes.

6.2. Clinical Use

In view of the less predictable response to subsequent doses when the drug is given for several days in succession,[41] we have limited our use of dDAVP to those situations in which it was anticipated that a short-term increase in F VIII would suffice. These situations included early acute hemarthroses in individuals with mild or moderate hemophilia A, and tonsillectomy, teeth extractions, and other oral or nasal surgical procedures in individuals with mild or moderate hemophilia A and vWD. We have continued to use the antifibrinolytic agent EACA for individuals with hemophilia or vWD who are undergoing extractions of permanent teeth, or any other oral surgical procedure. as an adjunct to treatment with dDAVP, just as we had done when blood derivatives were used.[1] On the other hand, we have not used EACA when dDAVP has been used for acute hemarthroses, despite the very brief increase in plasminogen activator that follows dDAVP administration.

6.3. Use of dDAVP for Menorrhagia

The two women whose severe menorrhagia seemed to benefit from dDAVP administration are of particular interest, in that menorrhagia is a real problem in many women with vWD. However, the efficacy of dDAVP in this situation will have to be evaluated in larger numbers of individuals before any conclusions can be drawn.

6.4. Selection of Subjects

While all individuals who have some measurable baseline F VIII activity will have an approximately threefold increase in F VIII activity following dDAVP, one must select those patients who are likely to benefit from such an increase in endogenously produced F VIII. In individuals with hemophilia A, this selection can be made on the basis of the person's usual baseline F

VIII:C value. Those with F VIII:C of 0.5–0.20 U/ml (5–20%) would seem to be ideal candidates for dDAVP whenever a threefold increase in F VIII:C of several hours' duration would be sufficient treatment.

Among vWD subjects, those with subnormal amounts of functionally normal F VIII molecules are likely to benefit. In those with severe vWD, with no detectable F VIII to start with, there will be none to be released from the storage sites, and thus no increase in F VIII. In those vWD variants in which abnormal molecular forms of F VIII:RAg are produced, F VIII components will rise following dDAVP, but they will still be the abnormal forms, which are often not hemostatically effective.[11] Thus, before administering dDAVP for a surgical situation one should determine which type of vWD an individual has. Whenever possible, one should also give a test dose of dDAVP several days preoperatively, to see if there is correction of the bleeding time with dDAVP.

7. SUMMARY

The vasopressin analogue 1-desamino-8-D-arginine vasopressin appears to be a safe and effective alternative to the use of blood products for individuals with mild or moderate hemophilia A, and in some individuals with von Willebrand's disease. This drug, when administered either intranasally or intravenously, results in a rapid two- to threefold increase in all components of the F VIII system. The rise is greater and more predictable when dDAVP is given intravenously, thus this route would seem preferable for dental extractions and other surgical situations. Patient selection is important, as not all will benefit from dDAVP.

8. ADDENDUM

Since the preparation of this manuscript, we have extended our observations with dDAVP in additional subjects with vWD and with mild and moderate hemophilia A. Our total experience to date (February 1984) includes 8 normal individuals, 60 subjects with vWD (type 1), and 20 with mild or moderate hemophilia A. All have had an excellent response to dDAVP, and no adverse effects were noted.

In addition to the patient studies we have also conducted in vitro experiments in an attempt to determine whether or not ddAVP has a direct
effect on the vessel wall. These studies, which utilized the human umbilical
vein model[48,49] and scanning electron microscopy, demonstrated that ddAVP
does have a direct effect on isolated vessel segments, with increased platelet
adhesion and platelet spreading at injury sites.[50]

The parenteral form of ddAVP was licensed for use in patients with
mild hemophilia and vWD in the U.S. in February 1984, and it is now
commercially available through Revlon-Armour under the trade name Sti-
mate®.

REFERENCES

1. Lusher JM: Hemophilia and related conditions, in Conn HF (ed) Conn's Current Therapy.
   Philadelphia, WB Saunders, 1981, pp 278–287.
2. Bloom AL: The von Willebrand syndrome. Semin Hematol 17:215–227, 1980.
3. Ruggeri ZM, Zimmerman TS: Variant von Willebrand's disease. Characterization of two
   subtypes by analysis of multimeric composition of factor VIII/von Willebrand factor in
   plasma and platelets. J Clin Invest 65:1318–1325, 1980.
4. Mikami S, Takahashi Y, Nishino M, et al: Heterogeneity of molecular size of factor VIII/von
   Willebrand factor in von Willebrand's disease. Thromb Haemostas 45:272–275, 1981.
5. Green D, Philip KJ: Variant von Willebrand's disease. A study emphasizing crossed-im-
   munoelectrophoresis. Thromb Haemostas 43:2–5, 1980.
6. Takahashi H: Studies on the pathophysiology and treatment of von Willebrand's disease.
   Thromb Res 21:357–365, 1981.
7. Ruggeri ZM, Pareti FI, Mannucci P, et al: Heightened interaction between platelets and
   factor VIII/von Willebrand factor in a new subtype of von Willebrand's disease. N Engl J
   Med 302:1047–1051, 1980.
8. Zimmerman TS, Abildgaard CF, Meyer D: The factor VIII abnormality in severe von
   Willebrand's disease. N Engl J Med 301:1307–1310, 1979.
9. Hanna W, McCarroll D, McDonald T, et al: Variant von Willebrand's disease and pregnancy.
   Blood 58:873–879, 1981.
10. Nachman RL, Jaffe EA, Miller C, et al: Structural analysis of factor VIII antigen in von
    Willebrand disease. Proc Natl Acad Sci USA 77:6832–6836, 1980.
11. Ludlam CA, Peake IR, Allen N, et al: Factor VIII and fibrinolytic response to deamino-8-
    D-arginine vasopressin in normal subjects and dissociate response in some patients with
    haemophilia and von Willebrand's disease. Br J Haematol 45:499–511, 1980.
12. Fukui H, Mikami S, Takase T, et al: Patterns of factor VIII related antigen on crossed
    immunoelectrophoresis and large pore polyacrylamide gel-crossed immunoelectrophoresis
    in von Willebrand's disease. Br J Haematol 46:269–276, 1980.
13. Myers TJ, Tembrevilla-Zubiri CL, Klatsky AV, et al: Recurrent acute hepatitis following
    the use of factor VIII concentrates. Blood 55:748–751, 1980.

14. Spero JA, Lewis JH, Fisher SE, et al: The high risk of chronic liver disease in multitransfused juvenile hemophiliac patients. *J Pediatr* 94:875–878, 1979.

15. Lesesne HR, Morgan JE, Blatt PM, et al: Liver biopsy in hemophilia A. *Ann Intern Med* 86:703–707, 1977.

16. Hilgartner MW, Giardina P: Liver dysfunction in patients with hemophilia A, B and von Willebrand's disease. *Transfusion* 17:495–499, 1977.

17. Spero JA, Lewis JH, VanThiel DH, et al: Asymptomatic structural liver disease in hemophilia. *N Engl J Med* 298:1373–1378, 1978.

18. Craske J, Dilling N, Stern D: An outbreak of hepatitis associated with intravenous injection of factor VIII concentrate. *Lancet* 2:221–223, 1975.

19. Seef LB, Hoofnagle J: Chronic hepatitis in hemophilia. *Ann Intern Med* 86:818–820, 1977.

20. Schimpf K, Zimmermann K, Rudel J, et al: Results of liver biopsies, rate of icteric hepatitis, and frequency of anti-HB_s and HB_s-antigen in patients of the Heidelberg hemophilia center. *Thromb Haemostas* 38:340, 1977.

21. Hruby MA, Schauf V: Transfusion-related short-incubation hepatitis in hemophilic patients. *J Am Med Assoc* 240:1355–1357, 1978.

22. McGrath KM, Lilleyman JS, Triger DR, et al: Liver disease complicating severe haemophilia in childhood. *Arch Dis Child* 55:537–540, 1980.

23. Preston FE, Triger DR, Underwood JCE, et al: Percutaneous liver biopsy and chronic liver disease in haemophiliacs. *Lancet* 2:592–594, 1978.

24. McVerry BA, Ross MGR, Knowles WA, et al: Viral exposure and abnormal liver function in haemophilia. *J Clin Pathol* 32:377–381, 1979.

25. Kim HC, Saidi P, Ackley AM, et al: Prevalence of type B and non-A, non-B hepatitis in hemophilia: Relationship to chronic liver disease. *Gastroenterology* 79:1159–1164, 1980.

26. Koretz RL, Stone O, Gitnick GL: The long-term course of non-A, non-B post-transfusion hepatitis. *Gastroenterology* 79:893–898, 1980.

27. Aach RD, Kahn RA: Post-transfusion hepatitis: Current perspectives. *Ann Intern Med* 92:539–546, 1980.

28. Vosburgh CH, Richards AN: An experimental study of the sugar content and extravascular coagulation of the blood after administration of adrenalin. *Am J Physiol* 9:35–51, 1903.

29. Marciniakøwna E: Wpływ adrenaliny na krzepliwosc krwi [Effect of adrenalin on blood coagulation]. *Acta Physiol Pol* 8:17–40, 1957.

30. Ingram GIC: Increase in antihaemophilic globulin activity following infusion of adrenaline. *J Physiol* 156:217–224, 1961.

31. Egeberg O: The effect of edema drainage on the blood clotting system. *Scand J Clin Lab Invest* 15:14–19, 1963.

32. Hawkey CM, Britton BS, Wood WG, et al: Changes in blood catecholamine levels and blood coagulation and fibrinolytic activity in response to graded exercise in man. *Br J Haematol* 29:377–382, 1975.

33. Mannucci PM, Aberg M, Nilsson IM, et al: Mechanism of plasminogen activator and factor VIII increase after vasoactive drugs. *Br J Haematol* 30:81–93, 1975.

34. Cash JD, Gader AMA, da Costa J: Release of plasminogen activator and factor VIII to lysine vasopressin, arginine vasopressin, 1-deamino-8-D-arginine vasopressin, angiotensin and oxytocin in man (abstract). *Br J Haematol* 27:363, 1974.

35. Mannucci PM, Ruggeri ZM, Pareti FI, et al: 1-deamino-8-D-arginine vasopressin: A new pharmacologic approach to the management of hemophilia and von Willebrand's disease. *Lancet* 1:869–872, 1977.

36. Mannucci PM, Pareti FI, Holmberg L, et al: Studies on the prolonged bleeding time in von Willebrand's disease. *J Lab Clin Med* 88:662–667, 1976.

37. Theiss W, Schmidt G: DDAVP in von Willebrand's disease: Repeated administration and behaviour of the bleeding time. *Thromb Res* 13:1119–1123, 1978.
38. Menon C, Berry EW, Ockelford P: Beneficial effect of deamino-8-D-arginine vasopressin on bleeding time in von Willebrand's disease. *Lancet* 2:743–744, 1978.
39. Schmitz-Huebner U, Balleisen L, Arends P, et al: DDAVP-induced changes of factor VIII related activities and bleeding time in patients with von Willebrand's syndrome. *Haemostasis* 9:204–213, 1980.
40. Warrier AI, Lusher JM: DDAVP—A useful alternative to blood products in mild hemophilia and von Willebrand's disease (abstract). *Blood* 58(suppl I):227, 1981.
41. Mannucci PM, Canciani MT, Rota L, et al: Response of factor VIII/von Willebrand factor in healthy subjects and patients with hemophilia A and von Willebrand's disease. *Br J Haematol* 47:283–293, 1981.
42. Simone JV, Vanderheiden J, Abilgaard CF: A semi-automatic one-stage factor VIII assay with a commercially prepared standard. *J Lab Clin Med* 69:706–712, 1967.
43. Zimmerman TS, Hoyer LW, Dickson L, et al: Determination of the von Willebrand's disease antigen (factor VIII-related antigen) in plasma by quantitative immunoelectrophoresis. *J Lab Clin Med* 86:152–159, 1975.
44. Allain JP, Cooper HA, Wagner RH, et al: Platelets fixed with paraformaldehyde; a new reagent for assay of von Willebrand factor and platelet aggregating factors. *J Lab Clin Med* 85:318–328, 1975.
45. Buckell M: The effect of citrate on euglobulin methods of estimating fibrinolytic activity. *J Clin Pathol* 11:403, 1958.
46. Mielke CH Jr, Kaneshiro MM, Maher IA, et al: The standardized normal Ivy bleeding time and its prolongation by aspirin. *Blood* 34:204–215, 1969.
47. Hillman CR, Lusher JM, Barnhart MI: Tests of platelet function: Technical points of clinical relevance, in Lusher JM, Barnhart MI (eds): *Acquired Bleeding Disorders in Children*. New York, Masson, 1981, pp 149–169.
48. Barnhart MI, Chen S: Vessel wall models for studying interaction capabilities with blood platelets. *Semin Thrombos Hemostas* 5:112–155, 1978.
49. Barnhart MI, Wilkins RM, Lusher JM: Platelet–vessel wall interactions: Experience with von Willebrand platelets. *Ann NY Acad Sci* 370:154–178, 1981.
50. Barnhart MI, Chen S, Lusher JM: DDAVP: Does the drug have a direct effect on the vessel wall? *Thromb Res* 31:239–253, 1983.

INDEX

215